THE MOST AFFORDABLE AIR FRYER COOKBOOK 2021

Easy Recipes For Busy People On a Budget

Table of content

Introduction

The air fryer doesn't look like a typical deep fryer. This kitchen utensil is much more like a small, sleek, self-contained oven that uses the convection cooking method. It uses an electrical element that heats the air in the fryer and then circulates it evenly around the food for cooking. As a result, this hot air quickly cooks the food in the deep fryer and brings out the well-cooked food that is evenly golden and crunchy on the outside, but the inside of the food remains moist and tasty.

With the air fryer, frying food is healthy. As? The air fryer requires only a small squirt of oil or no oil to cook your cook. You can easily cook french fries, chicken wings, onion rings and more and get crunchy foods without the extra oil. And, compared to baking and frying, air fryer foods, especially French fries, are more crunchy and don't dry out, making the food even more impressive.

Since the air fryer is small compared to the oven, it quickly circulates hot air around its fan which cooks the food faster. The air fryer takes less time to reach cooking temperature than an oven which may take 20 minutes or more to properly preheat and begin cooking. So if you need to prepare your meals quickly, you'll love the time-saving features of the air fryer.

The air fryer doesn't just fry. You can cook a lot more with it! The air fryer can also roast, grill, stir-fry, grill and bake, even cakes.

You can make fresh or frozen food or reheat leftovers. Use additional accessories for the air fryer such as cake pan, pizza pan, rotisserie rack, baking tray, steaming inserts to cook a variety of foods.

If you live in a dorm, share a house or have a small kitchen, you will certainly appreciate the small size of the air fryer. The air fryer comes in different sizes, but its small size can be the size of a coffee pot, which doesn't take up too much space on the kitchen counter.

Hence, the air fryer is easy to move or store. The air fryer is also useful for taking it on your travel adventures and placing it in your office kitchen to cook fresh food.

Most cooks don't like cleaning kitchen utensils, but with the air fryer it won't be a problem for you in any way. The air fryer only has a fryer basket and a pan to clean, which is dishwasher safe and takes a few minutes to wash after cooking. Also, the cooking basket or pan is non-stick, so the food usually doesn't stick and instead slides onto the plate easily

Before we move on, you may be wondering what exactly an air fryer is. Debuted in 2010, the air fryer is basically a kitchen appliance that fries without oil. Or, if necessary, as little oil as possible. It does this by circulating hot air quickly with a built-in fan, a process that creates temperatures high enough to mimic conventional frying. For this reason, air fryers can fry food without the risks of traditional oil frying - such as oil burns or fire damage - and can do so in a more systematic and controlled way.

Since an air fryer uses hot air, some may argue that it works the same way as a conventional oven. However, it must be remembered that the two devices produce different results, often due to their technological differences. While ovens apply dry air and heat directly to the plate and require longer cooking times, air fryers contain technology that quickly circulates air around the plate, resulting in faster cooking times and a more attractive appearance. more fried.

How to use an air fryer

Since 2010 there have been countless versions of the air fryer, often with different styles and mechanisms. That said, it's usually best to consult with your service provider when it comes to using it, and if you're looking to replace your current brand with another, how it differs from your new appliance. There are, however, some similarities:

Use the right attachment. Before anything else, clarify with the recipe which attachment you will need for the dish. Do you need a mixer? A grill? And extra pan? Make sure you have everything ready.

Remove the pan. While air fryers don't need oil to work, not using thick oil means a greater chance of some dishes sticking to the pan or basket. That said, you can lightly wet the pan with oil to prevent food from sticking or add parchment paper for a true oil-free alternative. However, removing the pan is essential.

Set the temperature. Whether you're using Fahrenheit, Celsius, or the amount of watts, make sure you set the fryer to the right temperature or power level, so it doesn't overcook or undercook your dish. Some air fryers also provide "modes" or cooking options for certain types of food such as French fries and pastries.

Set the timer. Once the temperature is finished, just set the timer as indicated in the recipe and let it fly. You can experiment a bit with this. Furthermore, you can also take the pan out every now and then to add other ingredients: or to check your cooking; all you need is to pause the machine.

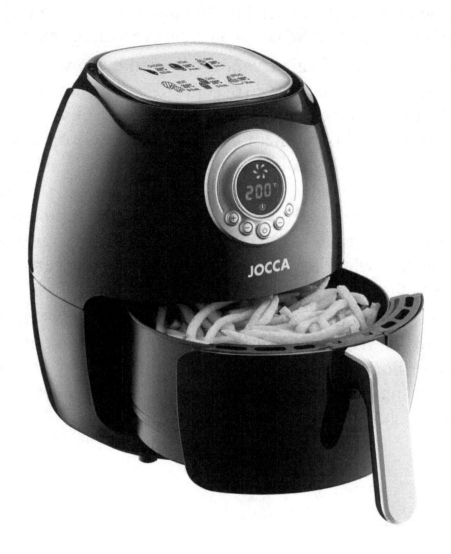

Chapter 1 The Air Basic Guide

Kitchen staples and spices from the pantry

My air fryer is an independent chef who takes the food I have prepared and turns it into a flavorful masterpiece. However, I still have to carefully select the best ingredients and spices to create mouthwatering dishes. Below are some of the cooking products and spices that I frequently use when cooking with my air fryer.

- **All-purpose flour**it's great for breading recipes, baking, and thickening sauces. All-purpose flour can also be substituted for healthier alternatives, such as almond flour, for those people who have special dietary needs.

- **sugar cane** it is the perfect ingredient to use in dessert recipes or in the preparation of sauces and marinades.

- **Butter**it is a great product to use for flavoring, but it can also be used as a fat. Both salted and unsalted butter work well in recipes. Be careful not to substitute margarine for butter as this could change the recipe results.

- **Eggs**they are used not only as the main ingredient (when making hard-boiled eggs) but are also used in dessert recipes or when making a washed egg for breading. You will find that all recipes call for large eggs.

- **Olive oil** will be used in most air frying recipes. It remains the healthier alternative to frying in cooking oil.

- **Bread crumbs** are the reason why air-fried foods are crunchy. You can choose between flavored or plain breadcrumbs (or season your own breadcrumbs at home).

- **Garlic**is one of my favorite spices to use when preparing meals. Make sure you have a bottle of minced garlic ready in your refrigerator! If you don't have fresh garlic, you can also use granulated or powdered garlic.

- **Sugar** it is an essential ingredient in most dessert recipes. White granulated sugar is the preferred option. Be careful when replacing sugar with honey as the flavor of the honey may change the recipe results.

- **Teriyaki sauce** is an absolutely delicious sauce to use as a marinade for poultry, seafood or beef. My favorite brand is Vay soy sauce and marinade.

- **Ground black pepper** it's a great spice to use when looking for another dimension of flavor without overwhelming food.

- **Salt** it comes in several varieties. The two main types I use are table salt and kosher salt. When I try to add a little more flavor (especially on meats), I will use coarse sea salt. Remember that since kosher salt and sea salt have much larger grains than table salt, you will most likely use a smaller portion in your dishes.

- **Mustard** adds a wonderful aromatic component to food. When harvesting mustard, you can choose standard yellow mustard or Dijon mustard.

- **Paprika** it is a great spice to use to prepare an egg or poultry dish.

Achieve the perfect time and temperature

There are so many factors that can affect cooking time, including the size, volume, thickness or temperature of the food. Factors such as power and humidity in the air can also affect cooking time. All of my recipes have been tested in 1,425 watt air fryers. This means that if your air fryer has a higher or lower power, the food may cook faster or slower.

For most recipes, the total cooking time shouldn't vary more than a couple of minutes, but to avoid overcooking, check your food regularly. A great trick is to check the food once you have reached the shortest cooking time displayed on the recipe. Determine if it is fully cooked or needs more time. Don't be shy about pressing pause and opening the air fryer drawer to check the food. This may save you from having to eat overcooked or burnt foods.

Eating raw or undercooked foods, such as eggs, meat, seafood, or poultry, can expose you to foodborne illness. The best way to make sure your food is ready to eat is to cook it at the perfect temperature. For example, lamb, minced meat, pork and veal should be cooked at temperatures reaching a minimum of 160 °F. Other cuts of meat, including beef steaks, need to be cooked to temperatures that reach at least 145 °F. All poultry, including turkey and chicken, must be cooked to temperatures that reach a minimum of 165 °F. The safest minimum temperatures for seafood can vary.

When reheating leftovers in an air fryer, reheat the food to a temperature of 350 °F and continue doing this until the food reaches a temperature of 165 °F. This is especially important when reheating potentially hazardous foods such as chicken, beef and pork.

Veggie Eggs and Cheese Cups

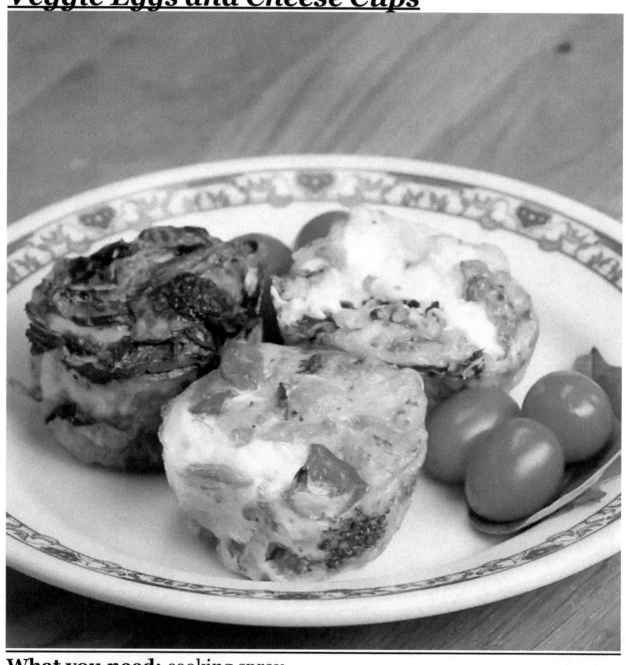

What you need: cooking spray
(olive oil) large eggs - 4 1/4 tsp.
salt 2 oz. half and half cheddar
cheese - 8 ounces, shredded
3 tsp. chopped cilantro

1/8 tsp. pepper

Steps:

1. Set the air fryer to 300 ° F to heat it up.
2. Spray freely 4 ramekin plates in glass or ceramic.
3. In a glass dish, mix half and half, salt, coriander, egg, pepper and 120ml. of grated cheese until combined.
4. Distribute the mixture evenly on the greased dishes. 5. Move the dishes into the basket in the air fryer for 12 minutes.

6. Once the time has elapsed, sprinkle the remaining 4 ounces. of grated cheese on top of each plate.

7. Set the temperature to 400 ° F and grill for another 2 minutes.

8. Serve immediately and enjoy your meal!

Useful tips:

You can add any of your favorites to these egg cups such as chopped veggies or extra cheese and customize them for different family members.

Store leftovers in a tub with a lid and refrigerate for about 4 days. When they're ready to eat, simply heat them for half a minute in the microwave.

_____

Egg-in-a-Hole

What you need:

Salt - ¼ tsp.

1 slice of toast

1 large egg 1/8 tsp.

pepper cooking spray

(olive oil)

1. Liberally spray the pan inside the air fryer with cooking spray.

2. Remove half of the slice of bread with a cookie cutter and move it to the pan.

3. Break the egg and place it in the center of the slice of bread.

4. Set the air fryer to heat to 330 ° F and cook for 6 minutes. 5. Use a metal spatula to flip the bread and steam for another 4 minutes.

6. Serve hot and enjoy.

French Toast Sticks

What you need:

1 tablespoon. cinnamon powder

4 tbsp. butter

1 cup of milk

5 large eggs

1/4 cup sugar, confectioner

12 slices of Texan toast

1 Teaspoon. vanilla extract Steps:

1. In a hot saucepan, melt the butter completely.

2. Meanwhile, cut the bread into 3 separate pieces.
   3. Using a glass dish, mix well the vanilla extract, melted butter, milk and eggs.
4. In another glass dish, combine the sugar and ground cinnamon.
5. Dip each slice of bread into the wet mixture and coat completely with the sugar mixture.
6. Transfer to a plate and blend the maple syrup and brown sugar.
7. Move to the basket of the air fryer and fry for about 8 minutes while setting at 350 ° F.
8. Remove the sticks from the air fryer and wait about 5 minutes before serving.

Useful tip:

Top your French toast sticks with your favorite toppings of powdered sugar or maple syrup.

_____

Ham and cheese omelette

Total preparation and cooking time: 15 minutes Ingredients: 1 protein omelette: 28 g.

Net carbohydrates: 5 g.

Fat: 18 g.

Sugar: 1 g.

Calories: 260

What you need:

Salt - 1/4 tsp.

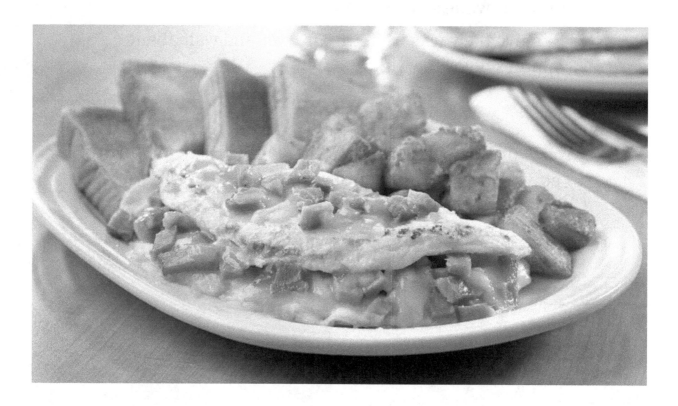

Milk - 2 oz. cheddar cheese -

1/4 cup, shredded

6 tsp. diced cooked ham

1/3 tsp. thyme dressing

2 tbsp. diced pepper

6 tsp. mushrooms

2 large eggs

1/3 tsp. seasoning of oregano

2 tbsp. onions, diced 1/3 tsp.

cooking spray paprika

dressing (olive oil)

1. Cover a 3x6-inch skillet with olive oil spray.

2. Beat the milk, salt and eggs until mixed in a glass dish. 3. Add the diced ham, pepper, mushrooms and onions and mix until combined.

4. Transfer to greased pan and move to air fryer basket.

5. Adjust the temperature of the air fryer to 350 ° F and heat for about 5 minutes.

6. In a glass dish, combine the seasons of thyme, oregano and paprika.

7. Open the lid and evenly sprinkle the toppings on top. Then sprinkle with grated cheese.

8. Steam for another 5 minutes. Use a rubber scraper to place between the omelette and the pan to lift. Transfer to a serving dish and serve hot.

Helpful tip: You can substitute mozzarella if you prefer instead of cheddar cheese.

Boiled eggs

Total preparation and cooking time: 20 minutes Ingredients: 6 eggs Protein: 3 g.

Net carbohydrates: 0 gm.

Fat: 0 g.

Sugar: 0 g.

Calories: 17

What you need:

6 large, cold eggs

4 cups of ice water Steps:

1. Adjust the temperature of the air fryer to 250 ° F and insert the wire accessory into the basket.
2. Place the chilled eggs on the grill and heat for 16 minutes.
3. Remove the eggs in a dish of ice water.
4. Once cooled, peel the eggs and serve immediately.

Home Fries

Total preparation and cooking time: 30 minutes Ingredients: 4 servings Protein: 1 g.

Net carbohydrates: 6 g.

Fat: 1 g.

Sugar: 0 g.

Calories: 53

What you need:

1 Teaspoon. salt

3 russet potatoes, cut into cubes

1 Teaspoon. chilli powder

3 tbsp. of paprika dressing

olive oil - 2 tbsp. pepper -

1/2 tsp.

garlic powder - 3 tbsp. Steps:

1. Adjust the temperature of the air fryer to 400 ° F to warm it up.

2. Prepare the potatoes by rubbing and cutting them into cubes.

3. Using a glass dish, combine the diced potatoes with the paprika, olive oil, chili powder, and garlic powder until integrated.

4. In a single layer, assemble the potatoes in the basket of the air fryer. Fry for about 25 minutes.

5. Open the lid about every 10 minutes to toss the potatoes so they are fully cooked.

6. Remove from the basket, arrange on a serving dish and serve immediately.

_____

Hash Browns loaded

Total preparation and cooking time: 55
minutes Ingredients: 4 servings

Protein: 5 g.

Net carbohydrates: 3 g.

Fat: 8 g.

Sugar: 1 g.

Calories: 246

What you need:

2   garlic cloves, minced

3   Russet potatoes

2 oz. chopped onions

1/4 cup red peppers, chopped

2 tsp. olive oil

1/4 tsp. salt

2 oz. green peppers in the cup, chopped

1 Teaspoon. paprika dressing

6 cups of cold water 1/8

tsp. pepper steps:

1. Rub the potatoes and peel them with a knife or peeler.

2. Use a grater to completely chop the potatoes with the largest holes available. Transfer the potatoes to a glass dish.

3. Empty the cold water into the pan and saturate for about 20 minutes.

4. Empty the potatoes and remove the moisture completely.

5. Set the temperature of the air fryer to heat to 400 ° F. 6. In another glass dish, whisk the potatoes, olive oil, salt, garlic powder, paprika powder, and pepper until completely covered.

7. Transfer the potatoes to the basket of the air fryer and steam for 10 minutes.

8. Open the lid and combine the onion, garlic and peppers in the basket. Mix the ingredients to be incorporated.

9. Heat for another 10 minutes and remove from the basket.

10. Wait about 5 minutes before serving.

Maple glazed bacon

Total preparation and cooking time: 20
minutes Ingredients: 2 omelettes

Protein: 28 g.

Net carbohydrates: 5 g.

Fat: 18 g.

Sugar: 1 g.

Calories: 260

What you need: brown
sugar - 3 tbsp. water -
2 tbsp. 8 slices of
bacon maple syrup - 2
tbsp.

Steps:

1. Adjust the air fryer to heat to 400 ° F. Remove the basket and cover the base with parchment paper.

2. Empty the water in the base of the fryer during preheating.

3. In a glass dish, beat the 2 tbsp. of maple syrup and 3 tbsp. brown sugar together.

4. Place the grill in the basket and arrange the bacon in a single layer.

5. Spread the sugar glaze over the bacon until it is completely covered.

6. Place the basket in the air fryer and steam for 8 minutes. 7. Remove the bacon from the basket and wait about 5 minutes before serving hot.

Helpful hint: If the sugar glaze is too thick, simply add a small amount of maple syrup to the desired consistency.

Biscuits with sausage, egg and cheese

Total preparation and cooking time: 45
minutes Ingredients: 5 biscuits

Protein: 7 g.

Net carbohydrates: 13 g.

Fat: 13 g.

Sugar: 3 g.

Calories: 190

What you need:

pepper - 1/8 tsp.

10.2 oz. can biscuits, flaky 1/8 tsp.

salt

1 1/2 tsp. vegetable oil

2oz. spicy cheddar cheese, diced into 10 pieces

1 1/2 large eggs

1/8 pound of
sausage, ground 1 1/2 tsp.

spray water for
cooking (olive oil)

Steps:

1. Create an 8-inch circle of baking sheeting and place it on the base of the air fryer basket. Cover with cooking spray. Place a separate piece of baking sheeting to the side.

2. Using a hot pan, empty the oil and brown the sausage for about 4 minutes, breaking it up with a wooden spatula.

3. Whip 2 eggs in a dish and blend with pepper and salt.

4. Remove the browned meat with a slotted spoon in a separate glass dish.

5. Set the temperature to medium temperature. Empty the egg mixture and heat for about 60 seconds, then add to the cooked sausage dish and mix thoroughly. 6. Meanwhile, cut the shortcrust pastry into 5 pieces and transfer it to the baking sheet.

7. Compress them in a thin circle and place a generous spoonful of meat and eggs in the center.

8. Place a cube of cheese on the filling and completely enclose by pinching the sides of the shortcrust pastry. 9. In a glass dish, combine the water and the remaining egg until smooth.

10. Apply the beaten egg to each of the cookies, covering it entirely.

11. Transfer to the basket with the sides pinched on the baking lining.

12. Set the temperature to 325 ° F and heat for 10 minutes. 13. Carefully turn the cookies over and continue to steam for another 6 minutes.

14. Remove the cookies on a plate and enjoy!

Sausage Patties

Total preparation and cooking time: 45 minutes Ingredients: 6 tartlets

Protein: 9 g.

Net carbohydrates: 1 g.

Fat: 17 g.

Sugar: 0 g.

Calories: 190

What you need: onion powder - 1/2 tsp.

11 oz. of sausage, ground and cold red pepper flakes - 1/2 tsp. thyme dressing - 1/4 tsp. salt - 1/8 tsp. paprika dressing - 1/4 tsp. garlic - 1 1/2 tsp, chopped brown sugar - 1 tsp. cayenne pepper - 1/4 tsp.

Tabasco sauce - 1 tsp.

Pepper - 1/8 tsp.

Steps:

1. Cover a baking sheet with the oven lining and place it in the basket of the air fryer.

2. Hand mix the cold ground sausage with all the seasonings listed, the Tabasco sauce and the brown sugar.

3. Divide the meat into 6 sections and make individual patties.

4. Move the meatballs into the basket in a single layer and adjust the air fryer to heat to 370 ° F.

5. Heat for 10 minutes and turn the meatballs on the other side.

6. Continue to cook for another 10 minutes.

7. Remove from the basket onto a serving dish and enjoy.

Helpful hints: If you prefer a spicier patty, season the meatballs with more tobacco sauce. Alternatively, you can substitute lean pork or chicken sausage in this recipe. If you don't have brown sugar on hand, you can substitute maple syrup.

_____

Salty bagel bites

Total preparation and cooking time: 30
minutes Ingredients: 6 morsels

Protein: 5 g.

Net carbohydrates: 23 gm.

Fat: 0 g.

Sugar: 1 g.

Calories: 130

What you need:

1 cup of self-raising flour

8 oz. Greek yogurt

1/2 cup cream cheese, whipped

cooking spray (olive oil) Steps:

1. In a blender, whip the yogurt and flour until it thickens into a dough for about 2 minutes.
2. Cover the base of the pan with cooking spray.
3. Make equal-sized balls of dough and transfer them to the greased baking sheet.
4. Close the top of the air fryer and adjust the temperature to 325 ° F for about 5 minutes.
5. Flip the balls over and reset to the same temperature with the Air Crisp setting for 4 minutes.
6. Remove the balls from the basket and let them cool for about 10 minutes.
7. Make a small hole in the sides of the bagels.
8. Pack the whipped cream cheese inside the holes using a pastry bag and serve immediately.

Helpful Tip: You can easily make a homemade pastry bag with a large ziplock bag. Add the cream cheese and slice the bottom corner with scissors. If you want a sweeter version, apply 1/2 teaspoon each of ground cinnamon and sugar to the balls after step 3. If you want them to be even sweeter, apply another 1/2 teaspoon each of powdered cinnamon and sugar during step 12.

Stuffed Baked Avocado

Total preparation and cooking time: 20
minutes Ingredients: 2 servings

Protein: 11 g.

Net carbohydrates: 3 g.

Fat: 6 g.

Sugar: 0 g.

Calories: 281

What you need:

> Two eggs, preferably large

Salt - 1/4 tsp.

> 1 avocado, large

parsley dressing - 3 tsp.

cheddar - 2 ounces, grated

pepper - 1/8 tsp.

Steps:

1. Set the air fryer to a temperature of 400 ° F.

2. Slice the avocado by cutting it in half and break the eggs into the hollow of the avocado.

3. Sprinkle the pepper, parsley, and salt on top of all the avocados.

4. Transfer the avocado halves to the basket and heat for about 14 minutes.

5. Remove to a serving dish and sprinkle with grated cheese before serving.

Sweet Potato Toast

Total preparation and cooking time: 40 minutes Ingredients: 4 servings

Protein: 28 g.

Net carbohydrates: 4.9 g.

Fat: 18 g.

Sugar: 1 g.

Calories: 260

What you need:

Salt - 1/4 tsp.

paprika dressing - 1/8 tsp. avocado oil - 4 tsp.

garlic powder - 1/8 tsp. 1 powdered sweet potato

onion - 1/8 tsp.

pepper - 1/4 tsp.

seasoning of oregano - 1/8 tsp.

Steps:

1. Heat the air fryer to 380 ° F.

2. Cut the ends of the sweet potato and discard it. Divide into 4 even pieces lengthwise.

3. Beat the avocado oil and all seasonings until well blended.

4. Brush the spices over the sweet potato slices.

5. Transfer the slices to the fryer basket and fry for 15 minutes.

6. Turn the sweet potato pieces and steam again for another 15 minutes.

7. Transfer to a serving dish and enrich with your favorite condiments.

_____

Tomato Mushroom Omelette

Total preparation and cooking time: 30 minutes Ingredients: 2 servings

Protein: 14 g.

Net carbohydrates: 4 g.

Fat: 14 g.

Sugar: 2 g.

Calories: 75

What you need: skim

milk - 2 tbsp.

pepper - 1/8 tsp. chives -

2

tablespoons, chopped

tomato - 1/4 cup, sliced egg

whites - 8 oz.

mushrooms - 1/4 cup, sliced Steps:

1. Adjust the temperature of the air fryer to 320 ° F.

2. Using a glass dish, blend the tomato, egg whites, mushrooms and milk until blended.

3. Incorporate the seasonings of chives and pepper into the mixture.

4. Empty into the pan and heat for about 15 minutes.

5. Serve immediately and enjoy hot.

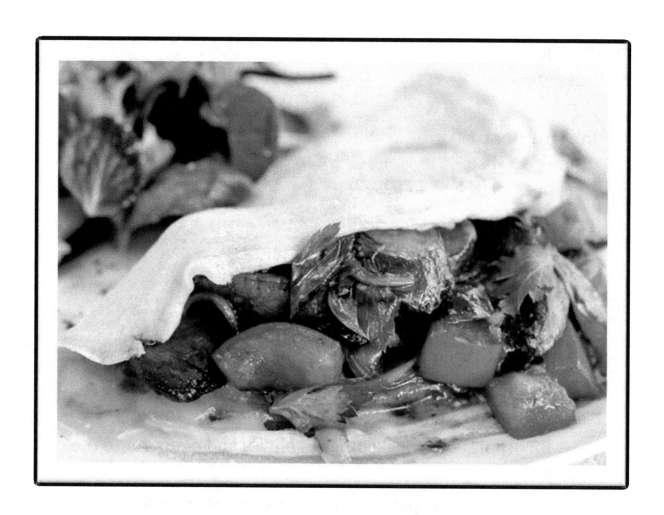

Bacon Cheddar Chicken Fingers

Total preparation and cooking time: 20
minutes Ingredients: 4 servings

Protein: 24 g.

Net carbohydrates: 6 g.

Fat: 26 g.

Sugar: 1 g.

Calories: 192

What you need:

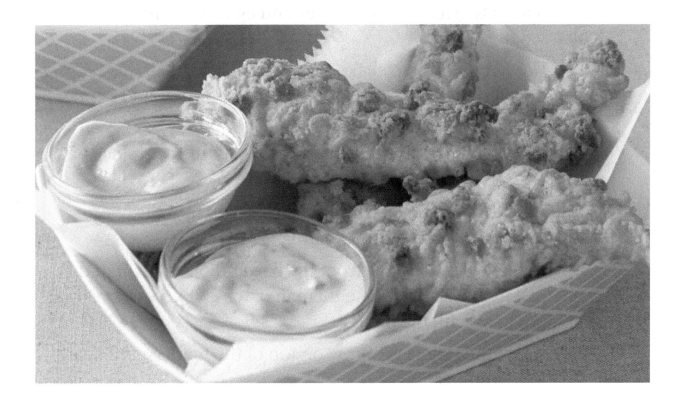

For the chicken sticks: 1 lb.
chicken tenders, about 8
pieces of spray cheddar
cheese

(canola oil) - 1 cup, shredded

Two large eggs

1/3 cup of bacon

2 table spoon. water for breading:

1 Teaspoon. onion powder,
panko breadcrumbs - 2 cups black
pepper - 1 tsp, freshly ground
paprika - 2 tbsp. garlic powder - 1
tsp. salt - 2 tsp.

Steps:

1. Set the air fryer to a temperature of 360 ° F. 2.
   In a glass dish, whip the water and eggs until well
   blended.

3. Use a zip lock bag, shake the garlic powder, salt,
   breadcrumbs, cayenne pepper, onion powder, and pepper
   together.

4. Dip the chicken in the eggs and shake it in the ziplock bag
   until it is completely covered.

5. Dip back into the egg mixture and again into the
   seasonings until a thick coating is present.

6. Remove the offerings from the bag and place them in the
   pan in the basket. Make them in batches if necessary so as
   not to overfill the pan.

7. Apply the canola oil spray on top of the tenders and heat
   for 6 minutes.

8. Turn the offers to the other side. Steam for another 4
   minutes.

9. Blend the pieces of bacon and grated cheese on a plate. 10. Sprinkle the bacon and cheese evenly over the hot tenders and fry for another 2 minutes.

11. Remove and serve hot.

Cod. In batter

Total preparation and cooking time: 30 minutes Ingredients: 4 servings

Protein: 35 g.

Net carbohydrates: 3 g.

Fat: 10 g.

Sugar: 0 g.

Calories: 371

What you need:

Cod - 20 oz.

Salt - 1/4 tsp.

all-purpose flour - 8 oz.

parsley dressing - 1 tbsp.

corn starch - 3 tsp. garlic powder - 1/2 tsp. Two eggs, preferably large onion powder - 1/2 tsp. Steps:

1. Whip the eggs in a glass dish until smooth and set aside.

2. In a separate dish, blend the cornstarch, salt, almond flour, garlic powder, parsley and onion powder, whisking to remove any lumps.

3. Dip the pieces of cod in the egg and then in the spiced flour, covering completely.

4. Transfer to the fryer basket in a single layer.

5. Heat the fish for 7 minutes to 350 ° F. Flip the cod and steam for another 7 minutes.

Useful tip:

Combine this fish dish with the French fries recipe and you have a Fish & Chips meal.

Beef skewers

Total preparation and cooking time: 30 minutes plus 1 hour of marinating

For: 4 Kabobs Protein: 23
gm.

Net carbohydrates: 4 g.

Fat: 15 g.

Sugar: 2 g.

Calories: 250

What you need: low-fat sour
cream - 1/3 cup of a bell
pepper
16 oz. of beef ribs, boneless
soy sauce - 2 tbsp. 6inch skewers -
8 pepper - 1/4 tsp.
medium onion - 1/2
steps:

1. Cut the ribs into sections about 1 inch wide

2. In a lidded bowl, combine the soy sauce, ribs, and sour cream making sure the meat is completely covered.

3. Refrigerate for at least half an hour, if not overnight.

4. Soak the wooden skewers for about 10 minutes in water.

5. Set the temperature of the air fryer to 400 ° F.

6. Slice the onion and bell pepper into 1-inch sections.

7. Remove the meat from the marinade, draining it well.

8 Arrange the onions, beef and peppers on the skewers and sprinkle with pepper.

9 Heat for 10 minutes, making sure to spin the skewers for 5 minutes during the cooking time.

10. Serve hot and enjoy.

Useful tips:

There are other cuts of meat that will work well for this recipe, including sirloin and beef stew.

_____

Cheese dogs

Total preparation and cooking time: 15 minutes Ingredients: 4 Hot Dog

Proteins: 12 g.

Net carbohydrates: 29 gm.

Fat: 13 g.

Sugar: 2 g.

Calories: 288

What you need:

4 hot dogs

1/4 cup cheese of your choice, grated 4 hot dog buns Steps:

1. Set the air fryer to heat to 390 ° F for about 5 minutes.

2. Place the hot dogs in the basket and cook for 5 minutes.
3 Remove and create the hot dog with the sandwich and cheese of your choice and return it to the basket for another 2 minutes.
4 Remove and enjoy while hot.

_____

Cheeseburger cupcakes

Total preparation and cooking time:
20 minutes Ingredients: 4 meatballs

Protein: 35 g.

Net carbohydrates: 0 gm.

Fat: 30 g.

Sugar: 0 g.

Calories: 425

What you need:

>   garlic - 1/2 clove,
>   minced ground beef - 1 1/3 cup
>   onion - 4 ounces, diced
>   Worcestershire sauce - 2 tbsp.
>   one egg, large
>   panko breadcrumbs - 2 oz.
>   cayenne pepper - 1/8 tsp.
>   cooking spray (olive oil)
>   salt - 1/4 tsp.
>   4 slices of cheese of your choice

1/8 tsp. pepper steps:

1 Using a large glass dish, combine the diced onion, pepper, chopped garlic, cayenne pepper, breadcrumbs, and salt until incorporated.

2 Blend the ground beef, Worcestershire sauce and egg and blend them carefully by hand.

3. Shape the meat into 4 individual meatballs and move them to the basket of the air fryer.

4. Coat the meatballs with cooking spray.

5. Set the temperature to 375 ° F and heat for 8 minutes.

6. Turn the burgers and steam for another 2 minutes.

7. Cover with a slice of cheese and continue cooking for about 3 minutes.

8. Enjoy it as it is or put it on a sandwich with your favorite toppings.

Helpful Hints: This is for a medium quality burger. If you prefer a rare or medium burger, heat for a total of 10 minutes. For well done, it will take a total of 15 minutes to cook.

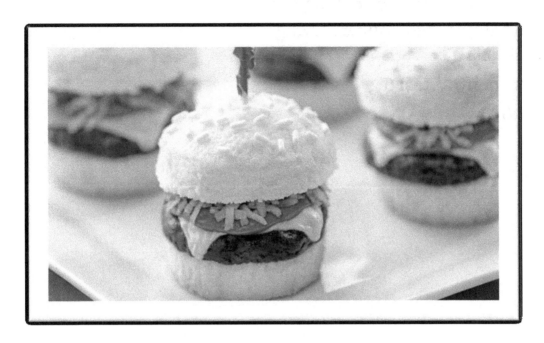

Chicken Cordon Blue

Total preparation and cooking time:
35 minutes Ingredients: 4 servings
Protein: 24 g.

Net carbohydrates: 6 g.

Fat: 26 g.

Sugar: 1 g.

Calories: 192

What you need:

Pepper - 1/4 tsp.
chicken paillard - 4 salt -
1/4 tsp.

Swiss cheese - 8 slices of all-
purpose flour - 1/2 cup Parmesan
cheese - 2/3 cup grated panko
breadcrumbs - 1 1/2 cup ham - 8
slices two eggs, large

Dijon mustard - 2 tbsp.

Grapeseed Oil Spray
Toothpicks Steps:

1. On a section of baking sheeting, brush Dijon mustard on each chicken paillard and sprinkle with pepper and salt 2. Place 1 cheese, 2 slices of ham and then the other slice of cheese on each of the chicken pieces.

3. Rotate the chicken starting on the longest side to create a roll. Secure in place with two toothpicks.

4. Whip the egg on a plate, empty the flour into a second plate and add the parmesan and breadcrumbs in a third.

5. Dip a chicken in the flour first, then dip it in the egg and then roll the chicken completely in the breadcrumbs. Press the cheese and breadcrumbs into the chicken to secure it and place it on a plate.

6. Repeat for the other chicken pieces.

7. Apply the grapeseed oil spray to each chicken section and transfer to the air fryer basket after 5 minutes.

8. Set the temperature of the air fryer to heat to 350 °. 9. Grill for 8 minutes and gently turn the chicken over to the other side. Heat for another 8 minutes.

10. Transfer to a serving dish and wait about 5 minutes before serving hot.

Helpful Tip: Alternatively, you can use Italian-flavored panko breadcrumbs to add more flavor to the recipe.

Sandwich with grilled cheese

Total preparation and cooking time: 10
minutes Ingredients: 1 sandwich

Protein: 17 g.

Net carbohydrates: 22 gm.

Fat: 8 g.

Sugar: 2 g.

Calories: 220

What you need:

2 slices of bread, softened

1   teaspoon. butter

2   slices of cheddar cheese

1. Set the air fryer to a temperature of 350 ° F.

2. Apply 1/2 teaspoon of softened butter to one side of the bread slice. Repeat for the remaining bread.

3. Create the sandwich by placing the cheese between the unbuttered sides of the bread.

4. Transfer to hot air fryer and let sit for 5 minutes. Flip the bun in half and remove it.

5. Serve immediately and enjoy.

Helpful Hint: Alternatively, add 2 slices of turkey or ham to this sandwich and cook for another 2 minutes.

Italian meatballs

Total preparation and cooking time: 35
minutes Ingredients: 3 servings

Protein: 24 g.

Net carbohydrates: 6 g.

Fat: 26 g.

Sugar: 1 g.

Calories: 192

What you need: one egg, large
        ground beef - 16 oz.
        pepper - 1/8 tsp.
seasoning of oregano - 1/2
tsp. breadcrumbs - 1 1/4 cup
garlic - 1/2 clove, chopped
parsley - 1 ounce, minced
salt - 1/4 tsp.
Parmigiano Reggiano - 1 oz. cup, grated   cooking
spray
    (avocado oil) **Steps:**

1. Whip the oregano, the breadcrumbs, the minced garlic, the salt, the minced parsley, the pepper and the grated Parmigiano-Reggiano until blended.

2. Combine the ground beef and egg into the mixture using your hands. Incorporate the ingredients carefully.

3. Divide the meat into 12 sections and roll it into slices.

4. Coat the inside of the basket with avocado oil spray to grease.

5. Set the temperature to 350 ° F and heat for about 12 minutes.

6. Roll up the meatballs and steam for another 4 minutes and transfer them to a serving dish.

7. Enjoy it as it is or combine it with your favorite pasta or sauce.

Helpful Tip: If you want to help with cleaning, simply cut a piece of baking sheeting to fit the base of your air pan. Have you finished the breadcrumbs? You can use a few slices of stale bread and crumble them in a blender.

_____

Loaded Baked Potatoes

Total preparation and cooking time: 25
minutes Ingredients: 4 servings

Protein: 24 g.

Net carbohydrates: 6 g.

Fat: 26 g.

Sugar: 1 g.

Calories: 192

What you need:

1/3 cup of milk

2 oz. sour cream

1/3 cup white cheddar cheese, grated

2 oz. Grated Parmesan cheese

1/8 tsp. salt to garlic

6 oz. diced cooked ham

2 medium russet potatoes 4
oz. sharp, chopped cheddar

1/8 cup. green onion, diced Steps:

1. Pierce the potatoes thoroughly with a fork a little while and cook in the microwave for about 5 minutes. Turn them to the other side and bomb them for another 5 minutes. The potatoes should be soft.

2. Use oven mitts to remove them from the microwave and cut them in half.

3. With a spoon, pull the inside of the potatoes about a quarter inch from the skin and spread the potato pulp into a glass bowl.

4. Combine the Parmesan, garlic salt, sour cream and white cheddar cheese to the potato dish and fully incorporate. 5. Distribute the mixture again on the emptied potato skins.
   Create a small cavity in the center by pressing with a spoon.

6. Divide the ham evenly between the potatoes and place the ham inside the cavity.

7. Place the potatoes in the deep fryer and set the air fryer to a temperature of 300 ° F.

8. Heat for 8 minutes and then sprinkle the cheddar cheese on top of each potato.

9. Melt the cheese for another two minutes, then serve with diced onions on top.

Useful tip: You can prepare them up to 5 days in advance and refrigerate until ready to fry. Simply cover with plastic wrap or store in a tub with a lid.

Stuffed Bell Peppers

Total Prep & Cooking Time: 30
minutes Makes: 2 Peppers Protein: 25
gm.

Net Carbs: 22 gm.

Fat: 5 gm.

Sugar: 1 gm.

Calories: 210

What you need: medium onion - 1/2, chopped
cheddar cheese - 4 oz., shredded pepper - 1/2
tsp. ground beef - 8 oz. olive oil - 1 tsp.
tomato sauce - 4 oz. Worcestershire sauce - 1
tsp. medium green peppers - 2, stems and
seeds discarded salt - 1 tsp., separated water -
4 cups garlic - 1 clove, minced **Steps:**

1. Boil the water in pot steam the green peppers with the tops
   and seeds removed with 1/2 teaspoon of the salt. Move from
   the burner after approximately 3 minutes and drain.

2. Pat the peppers with paper towels to properly dry.

3. In a hot frying pan, melt the olive oil and toss the garlic and
   onion for approximately 2 minutes until browned. Drain
   thoroughly.

4. Set the air fryer temperature to 400°F to warm up.

5. Using a glass dish, blend the beef along with Worcestershire
   sauce, 2 ounces of tomato sauce, salt, vegetables, 2 ounces of
   cheddar cheese and pepper until fully incorporated.

6. Spoon the mixture evenly into the peppers and drizzle the
   remaining 2 ounces of tomato sauce on top. Then dust with
   the remaining 2 ounces of cheddar cheese.

7. Assemble the peppers in the basket of the air fryer and heat fully for approximately 18 minutes. The meat should be fully cooked before removing.

8. Place on a platter and serve immediately.

Tuna Patties

Total Prep & Cooking Time: 20 minutes Makes: 4 Helpings Protein: 6 gm.

Net Carbs: 4 gm.

Fat: 2 gm.

Sugar: 0 gm.

Calories: 58

What you need: garlic powder - 1 tsp. tuna - 2 cans, in water dill seasoning - 1 tsp. allpurpose flour - 4 tsp.
salt - 1/4 tsp. mayonnaise - 4 tsp. lemon juice - 2 tbsp. onion powder - 1/2 tsp.
pepper - 1/4 tsp. **Steps:**

1. Set the temperature of the air fryer to 400°F.

2. Combine the almond flour, mayonnaise, salt, onion powder, dill, garlic powder and pepper using a food blender for approximately 30 seconds until incorporated.

3. Empty the canned tuna and lemon juice into the blender and pulse for an additional 30 seconds until integrated fully.

4. Divide evenly into 4 sections and create patties by hand.

5. Transfer to the fryer basket in a single layer and heat for approximately 12 minutes.

Helpful Tips: If you should have canned tuna packed in oil, it will work if you add an additional 2 teaspoons of almond flour to the mixture. This is also the case if the meat is too wet.

Banana Bread

Total Prep & Cooking Time: 50
minutes Makes: 4 Helpings Protein:
3 gm.

Net Carbs: 22 gm.

Fat: 6 grams

Sugar: 14 grams

Calories: 155

What you need:

all-purpose flour - 2
cups canola oil - 1/2 cup baking
powder - 2 tsp. four medium
bananas, peeled sugar - 2/3
cup, granulated sour cream -
1/3 cup two large eggs peanut
butter - 4 tbsp., creamy salt -
1/2 tsp. cooking spray (olive
oil)
walnuts - 1 1/2 cup, roughly chopped
vanilla extract - 2 tsp.
baking soda - 1/2 tsp.

Steps:

1. Adjust the air fryer temperature to 330°F. Coat the sides and
   base of a pan with olive oil spray.

2. Use a food blender, pulse the bananas for about 30 seconds
   until creamy.

3. Combine the sour cream, baking soda, eggs, peanut butter, salt, sugar, vanilla extract, and oil until thoroughly integrated for about 90 seconds.

4. Blend the flour and baking powder into the dough and pulse for an additional 30 seconds.

5. Using a rubber scraper, blend the walnuts until fully incorporated.

6. Empty into the prepped pan and smooth with the rubber scraper until even throughout.

7. Transfer the pan to the air fryer basket and heat for approximately 35 minutes.

8. Remove from the air fryer to a wire rack. Wait about 10 minutes before flipping onto a cutting board.

9. Slice into 4 equal pieces and serve warm.

Helpful Tips: Substitute Greek yogurt for the sour cream if you wish to have more moist bread. If you would rather have sweeter banana bread, you can alternatively use 3/4 cup of chocolate chips in place of the walnuts. The bread can be stored for 7 days in a lidded tub on the counter or for 3 months in the freezer.

_____

Chocolate Croissants

Total Prep & Cooking Time: 10 minutes

Makes: 8 Croissants

Protein: 2 gm.

Net Carbs: 14 gm.

Fat: 6 gm.

Sugar: 6 gm.

Calories: 110

What you need:

8 oz. can croissant rolls

1/2 cup chocolate chips **Steps:**

1. Open the can of croissant rolls and completely unroll the individual slices of dough onto a piece of baking lining. 2. Arrange a line of approximately 6 chocolate chips on the longer end of the dough and rotate into a roll.

3. Move the croissants to the basket of the air fryer and heat to the temperature of 320°F for about 4 minutes.

4. Flip the rolls over and fry for another 2 minutes.

5. Serve immediately and enjoy!

Corn Bread

Total Prep & Cooking Time: 35
minutes Makes: 4 Helpings Protein:
4 gm.

Net Carbs: 27 gm.

Fat: 5 gm.

Sugar: 2 gm.

Calories: 174

What you need:

Cornmeal - 1 cup

Sugar - 3 tsp., granulated

Butter - 6 tbsp., unsalted and
melted baking powder - 1 1/2 tsp.
all-purpose flour - 3/4 cup baking
soda - 1/2 tsp. Two eggs, large Salt -
1/4 tsp.

butter - 2 tbsp.,
unsalted buttermilk - 12 oz.

Steps:

1. Dissolve the 2 tablespoons of butter in a saucepan. Rub on
the inside and base of an 8-inch pan. Set the baking pan to the
side.

2. Adjust the temperature on the air fryer to heat at 360°F. 3.
In a glass dish, whisk the baking powder, sugar, salt, baking
soda, flour, and cornmeal until there are no lumps present.

4. Blend the 6 tablespoons of butter, eggs, and buttermilk into
the dish and completely integrate. The consistency will be
slightly lumpy.

5. Distribute the batter to the prepped pan and place inside the
air fryer basket.

6. Fry for a total of 25 minutes and remove. Slice after approximately 10 minutes and enjoy!

Garlic Cheese Buns

Total Prep & Cooking Time: 10 minutes Makes: 4 Rolls Protein: 2 gm.

Net Carbs: 16 gm.

Fat: 3 gm.

Sugar: 3 gm.

Calories: 112

What you need:

4 dinner rolls

1 cup your favorite cheese, grated

4 tbsp. butter, melted

1 clove garlic, chopped **Steps:**

1. Set the air fryer to heat at a temperature of 350°F. 2. Blend the butter and garlic in a saucepan and remove from the burner after approximately 2 minutes to cool.

3. Slice the tops of the rolls to create a large hollow. 4. Equally, divide the cheese between the rolls and pack into the indentions.

5. Brush the garlic butter on each roll, covering as much as possible.

6. Transfer to the air fryer basket and steam for approximately 5 minutes.

7. Remove and enjoy immediately while hot.

Hush Puppies

Total Prep & Cooking Time: 30 minutes

Makes: 12 Hush Puppies

Protein: 2 gm.

Net Carbs: 16 gm.

Fat: 3 gm.

Sugar: 3 gm.

Calories: 112

What you need: one egg, preferably large allpurpose flour - 3/4 cup cornmeal - 8 oz. baking powder - 1 1/2 tsp. onion - 2 oz., chopped salt - 1/2 tsp. milk - 3/4 cup sugar - 1/4 tsp.
cooking spray (olive oil) **Steps:**

1. Insert a section of tin foil on the bottom of the basket of the air fryer.
2. Blend the sugar, baking powder, flour, cornmeal, and salt in a glass dish until incorporated.
3. Combine the egg, chopped onion and milk into the batter and integrate well.
4. Section the dough into 12 equal portions by using a cookie scooper.
5. Create mounds out of each section and transfer to the air fryer basket.
6. Coat the hush puppies with cooking spray (olive oil) and heat for 10 minutes at a temperature of 390°F.

7. Open the lid and carefully flip the hush puppies over. Spray an additional time with olive oil spray and continue to fry for another 10 minutes.

8. Remove and enjoy immediately while hot.

Monkey Bread

Total Prep & Cooking Time: 15
minutes Makes: 8 Rolls Protein: 1
gm.

Net Carbs: 6 gm.

Fat: 8 gm.

Sugar: 2 gm.

Calories: 110

What you need:

self-rising flour - 8 oz. Sugar -
1 tsp., granulated non-fat Greek
yogurt - 8
oz. cooking spray (olive oil) ground
cinnamon - 1/2
tsp. **Steps:**

1. Using a glass dish, blend the flour and yogurt for approximately 2 minutes until it becomes a thick dough. 2. Section into 8 equal portions and form into small mounds rolling by hand.

3. Empty the cinnamon and sugar into a ziplock bag and shake the balls in the mixture until fully coated.

4. Coat the base and inside of a mini bread pan with the cooking spray (olive oil) and press the dough balls together inside.

5. Dust with the desired amount of the remaining sugar and cinnamon mix and heat at 375°F for about 7 minutes. 6. Remove from the air fryer and wait approximately 5 minutes before serving hot.

Potato Stuffed Bread Rolls

Total Prep & Cooking Time: 1 hour 20 minutes Makes: 8 Rolls, 4 Helpings Protein: 24 gm.

Net Carbs: 6 gm.

Fat: 26 gm.

Sugar: 1 gm.

Calories: 192

What you need:

- 1 cup coriander, chopped finely
- 2 small onions, chopped finely
- 5 large russet potatoes
- 1/2 tsp. turmeric seasoning
- 2 sprigs curry leaves
- 8 1/2 cups water, separated
- 2 1/2 tbsp. cooking oil, separated
- 1 1/4 tsp. salt, separated
- 8 slices bread, crusts removed
- 1/2 tsp. mustard seeds

2 jalapeno, seeded and chopped finely **Steps:**

1. Use a vegetable knife to peel the skins off the potatoes. 2. Warm a stewpot with 1 teaspoon of salt and 8 cups of the water. Once bubbling, adjust the heat to the medium setting.

3. Transfer the skinned potatoes to the pot and cover with a top. Steam the russet potatoes for approximately 15 minutes when they will be tender and remove from the burner.

4. Drain the water thoroughly and crush the potatoes completely with a masher.

5. Dissolve 1 tbsp. of the cooking oil in a hot pan and empty the mustard seeds into the pan. Blend the chopped onions into the skillet after approximately 20 seconds. 6. Sauté the onions for about 90 seconds and combine the curry leaves and turmeric into the pan.

7. Promptly distribute the mashed potatoes to the skillet and blend the remaining 1/4 teaspoon of salt.

8. Keep over the heat, occasionally stirring for about 60 seconds and remove from the burner.

9. After approximately 10 minutes, divide the potatoes into 8 sections.

10. Form oval rolls from each of the sections by hand and set to the side on a piece of baking lining.

11. Adjust the air fryer to the temperature of 390°F. Grease the inside of the basket with 1/2 tablespoon of cooking oil.

12. Using a glass dish, empty the remaining 1/2 cup of water on top of the crust- less bread.

13. Squeeze the individual slices of bread between your hands, keeping the bread flat, to remove as much moisture as possible from the bread.

14. Transfer one tablespoon of potato filler inside the moist bread and rotate the bread around to enclose the filling

totally while pinching the sides. Place on the piece of baking lining.

15. Repeat steps 17 and 18 for all 8 rolls.

16. Apply the remaining tablespoon of cooking oil on top of the rolls.

17. Arrange the rolls in the basket, so there is room for the air to circulate and heat for approximately 12 minutes. 18. Remove from the air fryer to a serving plate. Serve hot after about 10 minutes.

Helpful Tip: You can get creative with this recipe and substitute any filling into these rolls such as vegetables or meat.

_____

Pull-Apart Rolls

Total Prep & Cooking Time: 1
hour Makes: 6 Rolls Protein: 3
gm.

Net Carbs: 19 gm.

Fat: 2 gm.

Sugar: 4 gm.

Calories: 120

What you need:

> yeast - 1 1/4
> tsp. olive oil - 3 tsp. butter -
> 5 1/4 tbsp.
> pepper - 1/8 tsp.
> all-purpose flour - 2

cups whole milk - 1 1/8 cups coconut
oil - 3 tsp.

salt - 1/4 tsp. **Steps:**

1. Pulse the flour and butter in a food blender for about 45
   seconds until completely combined.

2. Blend the coconut oil, milk, and olive oil in a hot skillet for
   approximately 90 seconds and empty into the food blender.

3. Combine the yeast and completely integrate the dough by
   hand until it thickens for about 5 minutes.

4. Transfer to the air fryer set at a temperature of 140°F and
   heat for 15 minutes.

5. Transfer the dough from the basket and knead it for
   approximately 10 minutes.

6. Equally, section the dough into 6 portions and roll into a
   mound.

7. Arrange the bread balls so they are all touching into the
   basket. You do not need a separate baking pan. 8. Set the
   temperature of the air fryer to 365°F for approximately 15
   minutes and remove the rolls to a serving plate.

9. Serve hot and enjoy!

Helpful Tips: You may use your oven if your air fryer does not go as
low as 140°F for 20 minutes. This dough recipe can be used for any
type of bread or rolls that you would like to make including loaves.

Pumpkin Bread

Total Prep & Cooking Time: 45
minutes Makes: 6 Slices Protein: 3
gm.

Net Carbs: 37 gm.

Fat: 5 gm.

Sugar: 19 gm.

Calories: 140

What you need: ground
cinnamon - 1 tsp. sugar - 3
cups, granulated baking
powder - 1 tsp. pumpkin
puree - 15 oz.
can baking soda - 1 tsp.
olive oil - 8 oz. ground
cloves - 1 tsp. all-purpose
flour - 3 cups salt - 1 tsp.

three eggs, large
cooking spray (olive oil)

Steps:

1. Use a food blender to pulse the pumpkin puree, flour, salt, and eggs for about 60 seconds.

2. Combine the ground cinnamon, baking powder, sugar and canola oil and pulse for one more minute.

3. Finally, blend the ground cloves and baking soda into the batter for another 15 seconds until completely combined.

4. Cover the side and base of the pan with the olive oil spray.

5. Empty the batter into the prepped pan and adjust the air fryer to the temperature of 350°F.

6. Heat the bread for 35 minutes and remove from the air fryer.

7. Wait approximately 10 minutes before slicing and serving warm.

Finding this cookbook easy to use with a variety of useful recipes? We would appreciate your feedback in a review on Amazon.

Bacon Brussels Sprouts

Total Prep & Cooking Time: 45 minutes Makes: 6 Helpings Protein: 5 gm.

Net Carbs: 6 gm.

Fat: 2 gm.

Sugar: 3 gm.

Calories: 100

What you need:

- 1/2 lb. bacon
- 16 oz. brussels sprouts, cut in half
- 6 tsp. avocado oil
- 1/2tsp. garlic powder
- 6 tsp. lime juice
- 1 tsp. mint leaves, garnish
- 2 oz. pistachios
- 1 1/4 tsp. salt, separated
- 5 dates, pitted and diced
- 1 tsp. basil leaves, garnish
- 4 tsp. lime juice, separated
- 1/8 tsp. pepper

Steps:

1. Brown the bacon in a frying pan for about 3 minutes and set on a plate covered with paper towels.

2. In a glass dish, coat the brussels sprouts with 3 teaspoons of the lime juice, one teaspoon of salt, avocado oil, and garlic powder until completely covered.

3. Transfer to the air fryer basket with the temperature set to the 385°F.

4. Heat for a total of 25 minutes while tossing the brussels sprouts approximately every 5 minutes.

5. Crumble the bacon into a glass dish and set to the side.

6. At the 15 minute mark, combine the crumbled bacon, dates and pistachios into the basket of brussels sprouts and continue to cook for the remaining 10 minutes.

7. Remove and transfer the brussels sprouts to a serving platter and drizzle the remaining teaspoon of lime juice over the dish.

8. Dust the remaining 1/4 teaspoon of salt and pepper over the dish and garnish with the basil and mint leaves.

9. Serve right away and enjoy!

Total Prep & Cooking Time: 30
minutes Makes: 2 Helpings Protein:
9 gm.

Net Carbs: 40 gm.

Fat: 3 gm.

Sugar: 10 gm.

Calories: 221

What you need:

one large onion,
sweet salt - 3 tsp.

cayenne pepper -
1 /2 tsp. cooking spray
(olive oil) garlic powder
- 1 tsp. milk - 4 oz. one

large egg all-purpose
flour - 4 oz.
olive oil - 1/2 tsp. **Steps:**

1. You will need to prepare a piece of tin foil on top of a cutting board.

2. Brush 1/2 teaspoon of olive oil onto the center of the foil.

3. Slice the top half-inch of the onion off and remove the outer skin of the onion entirely.

4. Slice the onion in half, stopping half an inch above the root.

5. Make a similar cut perpendicular to the first, creating 4 sections of sliced onion.

6. Continue to cut the onion using this method and finish the cuts once there are 16 sections of onion slices.

7. Adjust the air fryer temperature to 370°F to heat. 8. Whip the cayenne pepper, garlic powder, flour, and salt in a glass dish with a whisk to remove all lumpiness.

9. Using another bowl, blend the egg and milk until combined.

10. Immerse the onion slices in the eggs ensuring they are completely coated.

11. Repeat by coating completely in the seasoned flour and spoon over each section to make sure no area is missed. Shake thoroughly to remove extra flour by turning upside down.

12. Apply the cooking oil onto each section of the onion and transfer to the air fryer basket.

13. Heat for approximately 10 minutes and remove if the crust is golden. If not, cook for an additional 5 minutes.

14. Serve immediately.

Helpful Tip: It is very important to leave half an inch uncut at the root of the onion. Otherwise, the sections of the onion will come apart during preparation.

Bok Choy Salad

Total Prep & Cooking Time: 10
minutes Makes: 2 Helpings Protein:
1 gm.

Net Carbs: 3 gm.

Fat: 0 gm.

Sugar: 0 gm.

Calories: 13

What you need:

> 1/2 tsp. sesame seeds, toasted
> 2 heads baby bok choy, halved

1 tbsp. toasted sesame oil

2 oz. shiitake mushrooms, stemmed

1/4 tsp. salt **Steps:**

1. Adjust the temperature of the air fryer to 400°F.
2. Slice the stems off the mushrooms and chop the bok choy in halves.
3. Apply sesame oil by brushing over the mushrooms and bok choy. Dust with salt and transfer to the air fryer basket. 4. Set for 5 minutes and remove to a plate. Drizzle the sesame seeds over the dish and enjoy while hot.

Cheesy Ravioli

Total Prep & Cooking Time: 25
minutes Makes: 15 Pieces Protein: 8
gm.

Net Carbs: 33 gm.

Fat: 3 gm.

Sugar: 4 gm.

Calories: 215

What you need: prepackaged ravioli - 16
oz., frozen bread crumbs - 1 cup
garlic powder - 3 tsp. parmesan
cheese - 1/2
cup two eggs, preferably large
Italian seasoning - 1 tbs.

cooking spray (olive oil)

Steps:

1. Blend the parmesan cheese, Italian seasoning, garlic powder, breadcrumbs in a glass dish.

2. Whisk the eggs in another bowl and set to the side.

3. Coat the basket of the air fryer with olive oil spray. 4. Immerse the frozen ravioli pieces into the egg making sure they are covered completely.

5. Coat the ravioli in the flour and transfer to the air fryer basket when breaded.

6. Adjust the air fryer temperature to 350°F and heat for a total of 15 minutes.

7. At the 8 minute mark, toss the ravioli to ensure they will fully cook.

8. Remove and empty onto a serving plate and enjoy immediately.

_____

Chicken Wings

Total Prep & Cooking Time: 30
minutes Makes: 4 Helpings Protein:
22 gm.

Net Carbs: 22 gm.

Fat: 19 gm.

Sugar: 17 gm.

Calories: 365

What you need:

pepper - 1 tsp.

chicken wings - 2 lbs. salt -

1 tsp.

sauce of your choice -3/4 cup

parsley seasoning - 1 tbsp.

Steps:

1. Using paper towels, remove the excess moisture from the chicken. Sprinkle with the pepper and salt.

2. Arrange the wings in the basket of the air fryer in a single layer so they do not touch.

3. Heat for 10 minutes at a temperature of 400°F. 4. Flip the chicken and continue to fry for an additional 10 minutes.

5. Use a meat thermometer to ensure the chicken is cooked to 160°F before removing to a glass dish.

6. Empty the sauce you have chosen over the chicken and coat the chicken completely using a rubber spatula to toss. 7. Grill the chicken once again in the air fryer at the same temperature for an additional 5 minutes.

8. Remove to a plate, sprinkle the parsley over the dish and enjoy hot!

_____

__Edamame__

Total Prep & Cooking Time: 10
minutes Makes: 4 Helpings Protein:
2 gm.

Net Carbs: 1 gm.

Fat: 1 gm.

Sugar: 0 gm.

Calories: 30

What you need:

> 1 tsp. avocado oil

16 oz. Edamame, unshelled and frozen **Steps:**

1. Drizzle the avocado oil over a dish containing the edamame and toss to coat completely.
2. Adjust the air fryer temperature to heat at 390°F for approximately 10 minutes.
3. At the 5 minute mark, stir the edamame.
4. Remove to a serving dish and enjoy while warm.

Helpful Tips: The edible part of edamame is the beans inside of the pods. It is not advisable to eat the pod, although you can if you prefer.

Eggplant Parmesan

Total Prep & Cooking Time: 45 minutes Makes: 4 Helpings Protein: 8 gm.

Net Carbs: 8 gm.

Fat: 4 gm.

Sugar: 8 gm.

Calories: 126

What you need:

eggplant - 1 1/4
lb. all-purpose flour - 3 tbsp.
parsley - 1 tbsp., chopped
bread crumbs -
4 oz. basil - 1 tbsp., chopped
parmesan cheese - 3 tbsp., grated
finely Italian seasoning - 1 tsp.
cooking spray (olive oil) salt - 1/4
tsp. marinara sauce - 8 oz. mozzarella cheese
- 1/4 cup, grated one egg white, large
water - 1 tbsp. **Steps:**

1. Slice the eggplant into half-inch rounds and sprinkle salt on either side. Transfer to a baking lining covered flat sheet and set aside for approximately 15 minutes.

2. In the meantime, blend the water, flour and egg white in a glass dish.

3. In a separate dish, toss the parmesan cheese, breadcrumbs, salt, and Italian seasoning until thoroughly integrated.

4. Adjust the temperature of the air fryer to heat at 360°F.

5. Using a fork to hold the individual eggplant slices, dunk into the dish with the egg and then the breadcrumbs, making sure not to over bread. Transfer back to the baking sheet.

6. Apply the cooking spray (olive oil) over the eggplant slices and arrange greased side down on a wire rack placed inside the air fryer basket.

7. Steam for about 8 minutes and open the lid.

8. Spread approximately a tablespoon of marinara sauce on each eggplant slice.

9. Divide the mozzarella cheese evenly and sprinkle on top of each serving of eggplant.

10. Heat for another 2 minutes and enjoy immediately while hot.

French Fries

Total Prep & Cooking Time: 30
minutes Makes: 4 Helpings Protein:
3 gm.

Net Carbs: 24 gm.

Fat: 7 gm.

Sugar: 1 gm.

Calories: 170

What you need:

salt - 1/4
tsp. olive oil - 2 tsp.
garlic powder - 1/4 tsp.
potatoes - 1 lb.
pepper - 1/4 tsp.

Steps:

1. Scrub the potatoes and remove the skins with a vegetable peeler if you prefer.

2. Slice the potatoes into long quarter-inch sections and place into a glass dish.

3. Using a rubber scraper, blend the salt, olive oil, garlic powder, and pepper over the potatoes, evenly coating. 4. Evenly arrange the fries in the basket of the fryer, keeping them 2 layers or less.

5. Heat the air fryer for approximately 20 minutes at a temperature of 380°F.

6. At the 10 minute mark, toss the fries gently and continue to broil for the remaining 10 minutes.

7. Empty the basket onto a plate and serve immediately.

Helpful Tip: If you like to have crispy fries, toss the potatoes again after cooking for 20 minutes. Then continue to fry for another 3 minutes.

Fried Green Tomatoes

Total Prep & Cooking Time: 20
minutes Makes: 4 Helpings Protein:
1 gm.
Net Carbs: 14 gm.

Fat: 7 gm.

Sugar: 3 gm.

Calories: 128

What you need:

Buttermilk - 1/2 cup

Two green tomatoes,
medium salt - 1/2 tsp., separated
two large eggs pepper - 1/4 tsp.
panko bread crumbs - 8 oz.

cornmeal - 1 cup all-
purpose flour - 4 oz.

cooking spray (olive oil)

Steps:

1. Chop the tomatoes into quarter-inch slices and use paper towels to remove the moisture.

2. Dust with the pepper and 1/4 teaspoon of salt on both sides and set to the side on a plate.

3. Empty the flour into a glass dish. In an additional dish, whip the buttermilk and eggs until combined.

4. In a third dish, blend the cornmeal and breadcrumbs.

5. Adjust the temperature of the air fryer to heat at 400°F.

6. Cover the slices of tomato firstly in the flour and then the egg, removing the excess.

7. Compress the tomato slices into the breadcrumbs on either side to help the crumbs to stick properly. Dust the tomatoes with the remaining 1/4 teaspoon of salt. 8. Coat the basket of the air fryer with the cooking spray and transfer the slices inside.

9. Apply a layer of cooking spray (olive oil) to the top of the tomatoes and close the lid.

10. Set the timer for five minutes and then turn the slices over.

11. Use the cooking spray (olive oil) to apply another coat to the tomatoes and continue to fry for an additional 3 minutes.

12. Serve immediately and enjoy while hot.

Fried Mushrooms

Total Prep & Cooking Time: 15 minutes Makes: 4 Helpings Protein: 0 gm.

Net Carbs: 0 gm.

Fat: 4 gm.

Sugar: 0 gm.

Calories: 44

What you need:

Salt - 3/4 tbsp.

baby portobello mushrooms - 1 lb. garlic powder - 3/4 tsp.

two eggs, large onion powder - 3/4 tsp. 1 tsp. creole seasoning, separated cooking spray (olive oil) panko bread crumbs - 1 cup pepper - 3/4 tsp.

all-purpose flour - 1 cup paprika seasoning - 3/4 tsp. **Steps:**

1.   Clean the portabella mushrooms by removing any dirt and slice into 4 sections.

2.   In a glass dish, whip the eggs and blend with 1/4 teaspoon of the creole seasoning.

3.   Empty the flour, garlic powder, salt, breadcrumbs, onion powder, pepper, paprika seasoning, and the remaining 3/4 teaspoon of the creole seasoning into a large ziplock bag. Shake until combined and set to the side.

4.   Transfer the sections of mushrooms in stages to the egg mixture. Once fully coated, shake to remove the excess egg.

5.   Transfer to the ziplock bag and agitate to coat the mushrooms completely in the breading.

6.   Remove the mushrooms from the bag and distribute to the basket of the air fryer, leaving space in between.

7.   Coat the mushrooms generously with the cooking spray. Shake the basket and spray the mushrooms on the other side with the cooking spray (olive oil).

8.   Adjust the temperature of the air fryer to 400°F and heat for 3 minutes.

9.   Open the lid and agitate the basket. Fry for an additional 4 minutes.

10.   Transfer the mushrooms from the air fryer to a serving plate.

11.   Repeat steps 6 through 10 as necessary.

12.   Serve and enjoy immediately.

Helpful Tip: You can also use white button mushrooms in place of the baby portabella mushrooms.

Total Prep & Cooking Time: 20 minutes Makes: 4 Helpings Protein:6 gm.

Net Carbs: 10 gm.

Fat: 2 gm.

Sugar: 0 gm.

Calories: 63

What you need:

one large egg salt - 1/2 tsp. okra - 2 1/2 cups allpurpose flour - 1 cup paprika seasoning - 1/2

tsp. cooking spray (olive oil) pepper -
1/2 tsp. **Steps:**

1. In a glass dish, whip the egg and blend with half the pepper and salt.

2. Empty the flour, paprika and the remaining 1/4 teaspoon of pepper and salt into a large ziplock bag. Shake until blended and set to the side.

3. Scrub the okra and dry using several paper towels to remove any moisture.

4. Remove both the ends of each piece of okra with a knife and discard.

5. Chop the okra into half-inch pieces.

6. Transfer the sliced okra in batches to the egg mixture. Once coated, transfer to the ziplock bag using a slotted spoon.

7. Agitate the ziplock bag to coat the okra completely in the breading.

8. Remove the okra from the bag and distribute to the basket of the air fryer.

9. Spray the okra with the olive oil.

10. Adjust the temperature of the air fryer to 400°F and heat for 4 minutes.

11. Open the lid and agitate the basket. Spray with olive oil once again. Fry for an additional 4 minutes. 12. Transfer the fried okra from the air fryer to a serving plate.

13. Serve and enjoy immediately.

Fried Pickles

Total Prep & Cooking Time: 20
minutes Makes: 4 Helpings

Protein: 3 gm. Net Carbs: 2 gm.

Fat: 2 gm.

Sugar: 0 gm.

Calories: 48

What you need:

> panko bread crumbs -
> 1/3 cup jar dill pickles - 16
> oz., whole one egg, large dill
> weed - 1/8 tsp. grated
> Parmesan - 2 tbsp.

Steps:

1. Drain the pickles from the jar and cut diagonally to be quarterinch thick slices.

2. Transfer to a few sections of paper towels to remove all the fluid.

   Set to the side.

3. Whip the egg in a glass dish and set aside.

4. Use a ziplock bag to shake the parmesan, dill weed, and bread crumbs until combined.

5. Immerse the chips in small quantities into the egg and shake to remove the extra fluid.

6. Transfer to the ziplock bag and shake until the chips are fully coated.

7. Move to the air fry basket and put no more than 2 layers of pickles in the basket. Repeat steps 5 through 8 for a second batch if necessary.

8. At a temperature of 400°F, heat the pickles for 9 minutes.

9. Remove and serve immediately.

Helpful Tip: This recipe is unique in that you do not need to agitate the basket halfway through. If you want to ensure the breading does not fall off, you can refrigerate the pickles after step 4 for approximately half an hour. You may also substitute pre-sliced pickles for the dill pickles.

_____

Grilled Pineapple

Total Prep & Cooking Time: 20 minutes Makes: 4 Helpings Protein: 1 gm.

Net Carbs: 54 gm.

Fat: 8 gm.

Sugar: 48 gm.

Calories: 295

What you need:

 butter - 3 tbsp. one small pineapple ground cinnamon - 2 tsp.

 brown sugar - 1/2 cup

Steps:

1. Dissolve the butter in a saucepan and empty into a glass dish.

2. Blend the cinnamon and brown sugar with the melted butter until combined. Set to the side.

3. Prepare the pineapple by cutting off the top and removing the outside completely.

4. Slice into several one-inch wide wedges.

5. Apply the sweetened butter to the sliced pineapple using a pastry brush and holding the pineapple with a pair of tongs.

   Alternatively, you can place them on a sheet of baking lining and apply the butter to one side. Then flip over the pineapple to apply butter to the other side.

6. Transfer the coated pineapple to the basket of the air fryer in a single layer.

7. Heat for 10 minutes at a temperature of 400°F.

8. At the halfway mark, open the lid and apply the remaining butter to the pineapple.

9. Remove the pineapple from the basket. It should have bubbling sugar on top.

10. Enjoy immediately.

Helpful Tip: If you have a smaller air fryer, you may need to do another batch. If this is the case, set the timer for only 7 minutes as the fryer will already be heated.

Kale Chips

Total Prep & Cooking Time: 15
minutes Makes: 2 Helpings Protein:
1 gm.

Net Carbs: 5 gm.

Fat: 2 gm.

Sugar: 0 gm.

Calories: 20

What you need:

salt - 1/4 tsp.

kale - 3 cups

cooking spray (avocado oil)

pepper - 1/8 tsp.

chili powder - 1/4 tsp.

Steps:

1. Remove the hard stems and tear the kale into smaller bitesized pieces.

2. Place the kale into the air fryer basket and coat with the avocado oil cooking spray. Toss to cover the kale evenly. 3. Sprinkle the salt, chili pepper, and pepper into the basket and shake again to coat the kale.

4. Heat for approximately 7 minutes at a temperature of 375°F.

5. Agitate the basket about every couple of minutes to make sure the kale does not stick.

6. Remove to a serving plate and serve hot.

Helpful Tip: You may use fresh kale or prepackaged for this recipe.

_____

Mozzarella Sticks

Total Prep & Cooking Time: 30
minutes Makes: 12 Sticks Protein: 3
gm.

Net Carbs: 2 gm.

Fat: 2 gm.

Sugar: 0 gm.

Calories: 48

What you need: onion powder - ½ tsp.

mozzarella string cheese - 5 oz. garlic powder - ½ tsp. cooking spray (olive oil)

one egg, large salt - 1/2tsp. panko breadcrumbs - 2 oz.

chili powder – 1/2

all-purpose flour - 2 tbsp.

paprika powder - 1/2tsp.

Steps:

1. Cut the mozzarella sticks in halves and transfer to a freezer safe zip lock bag. Freeze for approximately half an hour.

2. Whip the egg in a glass dish and set to the side.

3. Completely blend the garlic powder, breadcrumbs, salt, chili powder, paprika powder, and onion powder until integrated fully in a separate dish.

4. Prepare a flat sheet layered with baking lining. 5. Use another ziplock bag to combine the flour and mozzarella cheese by shaking until the cheese is covered fully.

6. Remove the cheese from the ziplock bag and dip into the egg fully and secondly into the breadcrumbs until completely covered.

7. Set on the prepped sheet and repeat for the other mozzarella sticks.

8. Freeze the cheese for approximately 60 minutes.

9. Adjust the temperature of the air fryer to 370°F to heat.

10. Coat the inside basket of the air fryer with the olive oil. 11. Remove the cheese from the freezer. Transfer 6 sticks to the air fryer basket and arrange so they are not touching.

12. Steam for approximately 5 minutes, remove to a serving platter and place the remaining cheese sticks into the air fryer basket for approximately 5 additional minutes. 13. Serve immediately with a dipping sauce of your choice or enjoy as is.

Nacho Chips

Total Prep & Cooking Time: 30 minutes Makes: 4 Helpings Protein: 2 gm.

Net Carbs: 16 gm.

Fat: 4 gm.

Sugar: 0 gm.

Calories: 130

What you need:

salt - 1/4 tsp.

sweet corn - 1/2 cup

all-purpose flour - 8 oz. chili powder - 1/2 tsp. all-purpose flour - 2 oz.,

separate water - 2 tsp.

butter - 3 tsp.

Steps:

1. In a food blender, whip the sweet corn and water into a smooth paste.

2. Combine the salt, chili powder, 8 ounces of flour, and butter and pulse until it becomes thick dough.

3. Dust the counter with the remaining 2 ounces of flour and flatten the dough with the use of a rolling pin until the desired thinness for the chips is achieved.

4. Slice into separate chips to your preferred size and shape. 5. Transfer the chips to the basket and heat for approximately 7 minutes.

6. Remove and serve with your favorite dip or salsa.

Onion Rings

Total Prep & Cooking Time: 1 hour 20 minutes Makes: 4 Helpings Protein: 20 gm.

Net Carbs: 79 gm.

Fat: 8 gm.

Sugar: 6 gm.

Calories: 506

What you need: two eggs, preferably large red onion - 13 oz. salt - 3/4 tbsp.
cooking spray (olive oil)
all-purpose flour - 2 cups pepper - 3 tsp.
panko breadcrumbs - 2 1/2 cups **Steps:**

1. Remove the outer layer off the onion and chop into thick ¾-inch slices. Take the rings out of the individual slices. Set to the side.

2. Create a dredging station with three glass dishes.

3. In the first dish, whip the eggs until smooth. In the second dish, empty the flour, and the third will contain the breadcrumbs.

4. Blend 1 teaspoon of pepper and 1/4 tablespoon of salt into each of the dishes and combine well.

5. Use a fork to immerse the rings individually into the egg dish and then the flour, repeating the process for finally covering with the breadcrumbs. Compress the breadcrumbs as necessary to help them to stick. 6. Make sure that each ring is covered fully but shake in between to remove the excess.

7. Place on a baking lining covered flat sheet and freeze for approximately 30 minutes.

8. Adjust the air fryer temperature to heat at 375°F. 9. Take the onions out of the freezer and transfer to the air fryer basket in a single layer.

10. Coat lightly with the cooking spray and fry for a total of approximately 12 minutes.

11. At approximately 6 minutes into frying, flip the rings over to the other side and spray again with the cooking spray.

12. Remove and enjoy hot.

Helpful Tips: You can pre-make these onion rings and freeze for up to 7 days. Alternatively, you can substitute other types of onions including Vidalia, Spanish or sweet onions. Avoid the yellow onions for this recipe.

Pigs in a Blanket Minis

Total Prep & Cooking Time: 45 minutes
Makes: 8 Pigs in a Blanket, 4 Helpings
Protein: 2 gm.
Net Carbs: 7 gm.
Fat: 2 gm.
Sugar: 0 gm.
Calories: 46

What you need:

4 oz. can refrigerated crescent rolls
8 smoked sausages, mini **Steps:**

1. Remove the moisture from the sausages by soaking up the water with paper towels. Set to the side.

2. Open the crescent roll can and flatten the dough on a piece of baking lining.

3. Cut the triangles into two equal pieces leaving you with 8 separate slices of dough.

4. Set a mini sausage at the longest section of the dough and rotate the dough to encase the sausage fully. Repeat this step for all the sausage links.

5. Transfer to the basket of the air fryer and heat at a temperature of 330°F for approximately 8 minutes.

6. Remove and enjoy as is or with your favorite sauce or dip.

Potato Chips

Total Prep & Cooking Time: 20
minutes Makes: 4 Helpings Protein:
4 gm.

Net Carbs: 17 gm.

Fat: 2 gm.

Sugar: 3 gm.

Calories: 86

What you need:

>   1 large russet potato cooking
> spray (olive oil)

3/4 tbsp. salt **Steps:**

1. Use a cheese grater or a kitchen mandolin to cut the potato into at least ¼-inch thin slices. If you can, make them as thin as 1/16-inch thin.

2. Soak up the moisture in the chips with several paper towels.

3. Coat the air fryer basket with the cooking spray (olive oil) and arrange a single layer of potato chips inside. 4. Lightly apply the top of the chips with additional cooking spray (olive oil).

5. Heat at a temperature of 450°F for approximately 15 minutes.

6. Remove to the counter on a platter and repeat steps 9 through 11 until all chips are complete.

Helpful Tip: The chips will get crisper if you leave them overnight on the counter. If you want to flavor your chips, dust the seasonings of your choice on the chips after you have sprayed with the cooking oil.

If you want them to be completely coated in flavor, toss the chips in a bowl with 1 tsp. of oil with the spices before transferring to the air fryer basket.

Pretzel Poppers

Total Prep & Cooking Time: 45
minutes Makes: 5 Helpings Protein:
1 gm.

Net Carbs: 3 gm.

Fat: 2 gm.

Sugar: 1 gm.

Calories: 25

What you need: Water - 4 cups butter - 2 tbsp.,
unsalted four-count refrigerated
buttermilk biscuits garlic powder - 1/4
tsp. cooking spray (olive oil) baking soda - 1/4
cup sea salt - 1 tbsp. **Steps:**

1. Prepare a flat sheet with a rim covered with baking lining. Set to the side.

2 Warm the baking soda and water in a big pot, bringing to a simmer.

3. Open the can of biscuits and slice into quarters, making a total of 20 pieces.

4. Create small balls and transfer to the simmering water for 2 minutes while occasionally stirring.

5. With a slotted spoon, scoop out the cooked balls and move to the prepped flat sheet. Let them cool for approximately 10 minutes.

6. In the meantime, liquefy the butter in a saucepan. Empty into a dish to combine with the garlic powder until integrated.

7. Adjust the air fryer temperature to 400°F.

8. Spread the spiced butter on each pretzel with a pastry brush.

9. Arrange the pretzels inside the basket in a single layer. Make sure there is space in between each ball. You will most likely need to fry in stages.

10. Set the timer for 10 minutes and turn the pretzels over at the halfway mark.

11. Remove to a serving plate and dust with the sea salt.

12. Repeat steps 15 through 17 until all pretzel bites are complete and enjoy!

Helpful Tips: Avoid using the flaky type of refrigerated biscuits in this recipe, as they will not stay in a uniform ball.

Rib Bites

Total Prep & Cooking Time: 25 minutes in addition to 2 hours of marinating time

Makes: 4 Helpings

Protein: 3 gm.

Net Carbs: 2 gm.

Fat: 2 gm.

Sugar: 0 gm.

Calories: 48

What you need:

pork riblets - 1 lb.

soy sauce - 2 1/3

tbsp. dry sherry - 3 tbsp.

sugar - 1 1/2 tbsp., granulated

garlic - 6 large cloves, peeled and halved

oyster sauce - 1 tbsp. **Steps:**

1. Slice the ribs into small half-inch pieces with the bone intact and transfer to a big lidded tub.

2. Blend the soy sauce, oyster sauce, dry sherry, sugar and halved cloves of garlic into the tub.

3. Cover the ribs completely in the fluid.

4. Refrigerate for a minimum of 2 hours if not overnight to marinate.

5. When the meat is marinated, heat the air fryer to the temperature of 360°F.

6. Remove the marinade from the fridge and drain extremely well.

7. Arrange the rib bites in a single layer in the basket of the air fryer, allowing for a room in between.

8. Fry for a total of 12 minutes while flipping the ribs at the halfway mark.

9 Remove to a platter and enjoy immediately.

Roasted Asparagus

Total Prep & Cooking Time: 10
minutes Makes: 4 Helpings Protein:
4 gm.

Net Carbs: 2 gm.

Fat: 4 gm.

Sugar: 0 gm.

Calories: 53

What you need:

> pepper - 1/8 tsp.
> extra virgin olive oil - 1
> tbsp. salt - 1/8 tsp.
>> asparagus - 1 lb.

Steps:

1. Slice the last inch of the base of the vegetables off and toss in the trash.

2. Transfer the cut asparagus into a dish. Empty the oil completely over the dish. Dust with pepper and salt. 3. Use a rubber scraper to cover the seasoning and oil over the asparagus completely.

4. Empty the asparagus into the air fryer basket and close the lid.

   Heat for 7 minutes at a temperature of 400°F.

5. Remove to a serving platter and immediately enjoy.

__Roasted Garlic Potatoes__

Total Prep & Cooking Time: 40
minutes Makes: 6 Helpings Protein:
1 gm.

Net Carbs: 54 gm.

Fat: 8 gm.

Sugar: 48 gm.

Calories: 295

What you need: oregano
     seasoning - 1/2 tsp.
   butter - 2 tbsp., unsalted pepper -
   1/4 tsp.
   garlic - 5 cloves,
   minced basil seasoning - 1/2
   tsp.
   red potatoes - 3 lbs.
   thyme seasoning - 1
   tsp. olive oil - 2 tbsp.
   parmesan cheese - 1/3 cup,
   grated parsley leaves - 2 tbsp.
   salt - 1/4 tsp.

Steps:

1. Dissolve the butter in a hot pot and move away from the burner. Set to the side.

2. Thoroughly wash and scrub the potatoes and chop into 4 sections.

   3 Use a ziplock bag to shake the basil, garlic, oregano, parsley leaves, salt, thyme, and pepper until thoroughly mixed. 4. Finally, blend the potatoes, melted butter, parmesan cheese and olive in the bag and agitate until the potatoes are entirely covered.

5. Cut a piece of baking lining to fit the base of the basket of the air fryer.

6. Empty the spiced potatoes into the basket and heat for approximately 20 minutes at a temperature of 400°F.

7. Stir the contents about 10 minutes into frying.

8. Remove to a serving dish and enjoy while hot.

Spiced Butternut Squash

Total Prep & Cooking Time: 30
minutes Makes: 4 Helpings Protein:
1 gm.

Net Carbs: 14 gm.

Fat: 7 gm.

Sugar: 3 gm.

Calories: 128

What you need: ground cloves - 1/4
        tsp. ground cinnamon - 1 1/2
        tsp. butternut squash - 4
        cups, cubed ground nutmeg -

1/2 tsp. ground allspice - 1/4
tsp. brown sugar - 2 tbsp.

ground ginger - 1/2 tsp.

olive oil - 2 tbsp. **Steps:**

1. Wash the butternut squash and chop into 1-inch cubes. Transfer to a glass dish.

2. Blend the brown sugar, cinnamon, nutmeg, allspice, cloves, ginger, and the olive oil until the squash is evenly covered.

3. Empty the dish into the air fryer basket. Adjust the temperature to 400°F and heat for about 15 minutes.

4. Shake the basket at the 8-minute mark and continue to cook until evenly browned.

5. Remove from the basket and enjoy immediately.

_____

Sweet Potato Tots

Total Prep & Cooking Time: 25 minutes

Makes: 4 Helpings, 6 Tots per Helping

Protein: 1 gm.

Net Carbs: 13 gm.

Fat: 4 gm.

Sugar: 8 gm.

Calories: 100

What you need:

     1/2 tsp. coriander seasoning

     2 cups sweet potato puree

     1/2 tsp. salt

4 oz. panko breadcrumbs

1/2 tsp. cumin seasoning
olive oil
cooking oil **Steps:**

1. Prepare a baking lining covered flat sheet and set to the side.

2. In a big glass dish, blend the coriander, sweet potato puree, salt, breadcrumbs, and cumin until thoroughly combined.

3. Heat the air fryer to the temperature of 390°F. 4.
    Spoon out approximately one tablespoon of sweet potatoes and create the shape of tots that you prefer by hand.

5. There will be 24 individual tots when you are finished and transfer to the prepped flat sheet.

6. Apply the cooking spray (olive oil) to the top and roll them around to apply to the bottom as well.

7. Distribute the tots to the basket of the air fryer in a single layer leaving room in between.

8. Set the timer for approximately 7 minutes and turn the tots to the other side.

9. Continue to fry for an additional 5 minutes.

10. Repeat steps 18 through 20 for the remaining tots.

11. Enjoy immediately with your favorite sauce or dip.

Helpful Tip: When you go to turn the tots, if they are soft keep them in for an additional 3 minutes before attempting to flip again. You can prepare these tots up to 7 days in advance and freeze until you are prepared to eat them. Simply move them to a freezer safe zip lock bag after forming the tots and label with the date. To heat, after they have been frozen, adjust the air fryer to the same temperature and cook for 10 minutes before turning. Then continue to fry for another 5 minutes.

Zucchini Corn Fritters

Total Prep & Cooking Time: 35
minutes Makes: 4 Helpings
Protein: 3 gm. Net Carbs: 2 gm.

Fat: 2 gm.

Sugar: 0 gm.

Calories: 48

What you need:

salt - 1/4 tsp.
one medium potato
cooked two medium
zucchinis garlic - 1 clove,
minced finely corn kernels - 8
oz.
all-purpose flour - 2

tbsp. olive oil - 2 tsp. Pepper

- 1/4 tsp. cold water - 3 cups

Steps:

1. Prepare a flat sheet by layering baking lining over the top.
    Set to the side.

2. Thoroughly wash and scrub the zucchini and potato. 3.
    Use a cheese grater to slice the zucchini using the largest holes and transfer to a glass dish.

4. Dust with 1/4 tsp. of the salt and let it sit for approximately 15 minutes.

5. In the meantime, nuke the potato for about 3 minutes in the microwave. Use oven mitts to remove to a glass dish with the cold water for approximately 5 minutes. 6.
    Remove the water from the bowl and use a vegetable peeler to remove the skins.

7. Replace the cooked potato in the glass dish and smash with a fork or masher.

8. Remove the extra moisture from the zucchini by twisting in a tea towel.

9. Using a food blender, pulse the zucchini, flour, salt, mashed potato, corn, and pepper for approximately 2 minutes until combined totally.

10. Adjust the temperature of the air fryer to heat at 360°F.

11. Spoon about 2 tablespoons of the batter and form into patties by hand.

12. Transfer the patties to the prepped flat sheet. Repeat until you have a total of 4 patties.

13. Apply the olive oil to the top of the patties using a pastry brush.

14. Arrange the patties in the air fryer basket, leaving space in between, and fry for 8 minutes.

15. Flip the patties over and continue to fry for approximately 4 additional minutes.

16. Repeat steps 19 and 20 if you could not fit the 4 patties in one time.

17. Serve while still hot and enjoy!

Helpful tips: Make sure that the zucchini is not bruised and is properly fresh and firm. You can easily use frozen or canned corn for this recipe.

Beef and Vegetable Stir Fry

Total Prep & Cooking Time: 50
minutes Makes: 2 Helpings Protein:
2 gm.

Net Carbs: 10 gm.

Fat: 7 gm.

Sugar: 0 gm.

Calories: 122

What you need:

For the stir-fry:

one yellow
pepper beef sirloin - 16
oz. one green pepper
onion - 1/2 cup broccoli
- 24 oz., florets one red
pepper red onion - 1/2
cup

1 tbsp. olive oil *For the
sauce:*

hoisin sauce -
1/4 cup sesame oil - 1
tsp. water - 1/4 cup
soy sauce - 3 tsp.
ground ginger - 1 tsp.

garlic - 2 tsp., minced

Steps:

1. Chop the peppers and onions into long strips and set to the
    side in a glass dish.

2. Slice the beef sirloin into strips approximately two inches long and set aside along with the vegetables.

3. In a lidded tub, blend the water, ground ginger, soy sauce, sesame oil, minced garlic, and hoisin sauce until thoroughly combined.

4. Transfer the sliced sirloin into the marinade and refrigerate for approximately 20 minutes.

5. About 10 minutes before you start cooking, heat the air fryer to the temperature of 200°F.

6. Drizzle the olive oil over the sliced vegetables and toss until covered.

7. Transfer the vegetables to the basket of the air fryer and fry for approximately 5 minutes.

8. Meanwhile, thoroughly drain the marinade from the sirloin.

9. Check the softness of the vegetables. If they are still hard, fry for another 2 minutes.

10. Transfer the air-fried vegetables to a glass bowl and adjust the temperature to 360°F.

11. Transfer the drained sirloin into the air fryer basket and heat for 4 minutes.

12. Flip the meat to the other side. Steam for approximately 2 minutes or to your desired level of doneness. 13. Remove to the same dish as the vegetables and serve immediately.

Total Prep & Cooking Time: 1
hour Makes: 2 helpings Protein:
23 gm.

Net Carbs: 4 gm.

Fat: 15 gm.

Sugar: 2 gm.

Calories: 250

What you need: beef fillet -
16 oz.

salt - 1/4 tsp.

olive oil - 1 tsp. puff
pastry - 10 oz. liver pate -
3.50

oz. two egg yolks pepper-
1/4 tsp.

Steps:

1. Heat a skillet to be very warm. Divide the beef fillet into equal halves. Apply the olive oil to the beef fillets with a pastry brush and sear the meat for about 30 seconds.

2. Turn to the other side and fry for another 30 seconds.

3. Remove from the burner to a plate and set to the side.

4. Whip the egg yolks in a small dish and set to the side. 5. Slice 2 puff pastries to be approximately 4" longer than the length of the fillets.

6. Apply the liver pate over the fillets and arrange in the middle of the individual pastries.

7. Rotate the puff pastry over the fillets, completely encasing the meat.

8. Remove the excess pastry and close the ends by applying the egg yolks with a pastry brush. Compress the ends together to seal properly.

9. Continue to apply egg yolks to the open sections of the pastry and seal them by pressing on the ends.

10. Move the encased fillets to the grill tray. Coat the top of the pastries with additional egg yolk and store in the fridge for 20 minutes.

11. Adjust the temperature of the air fryer to 350°F and remove the pastries from the refrigerator.

12. Slice the tops of the pastries about 4 times so they pastries will properly cook.

13. Fry for half an hour and wait about 10 minutes before serving hot.

————————————

Chicken Parmesan

Total Prep & Cooking Time: 20 minutes Makes: 4 Helpings Protein: 24 gm.

Net Carbs: 6 gm.

Fat: 26 gm.

Sugar: 1 gm.

Calories: 192

What you need:

Asiago cheese - 1/2 cup, grated 4 chicken breast paillards pepper - 1/3 tsp. one cup of milk panko bread crumbs - 4 oz. salt - 1/3 tsp. cooking spray (olive oil) parmesan cheese - 1/2 cup, grated

Steps:

1. Immerse the flattened chicken in a glass bowl with the pepper, milk, and salt for approximately 10 minutes.

2. Coat the air fryer basket with the cooking spray (olive oil) and heat the air fryer to the temperature of 400°F.

3. In an additional dish, blend the parmesan cheese, breadcrumbs, and Asiago cheese.

4. Transfer the chicken breasts to the breadcrumb mixture and compress the crumbs to ensure they stick.

5. Move 2 chicken breasts to the basket of the hot air fryer and apply the cooking spray to the top of the chicken. You will need to do another stage with the remaining chicken breasts.

6. Heat for 4 minutes and turn the chicken over. Spray again with the cooking spray and continue to fry for another 4 minutes.

7. Remove to a plate and repeat steps 16 and 17 for the other 2 chicken breasts.

8. When you have removed the last two breasts, replace the original 2 chicken breasts into the fryer for approximately 60 seconds to warm them.

9. Enjoy immediately.

Helpful Tip: You can use a combination of any type of any hard cheese that has been grated such as Romano cheese. You will need 1 cup of the combination of cheese(s).

Coconut Shrimp

Total Prep & Cooking Time: 25
minutes Makes: 4 Helpings Protein:
13 gm.
Net Carbs: 16 gm.
Fat: 6 gm.
Sugar: 7 gm.
Calories: 191

What you need: cornstarch -
1/4 cup two large egg
whites salt - 1 tsp.
large raw shrimp - 1/2 lb.
coconut flakes - 8 oz., sweetened **Steps:**

1. Blend the cornstarch and salt in a glass dish. In another dish, empty the egg whites. In a final dish, pour the coconut.

2. Use a fork to dredge the shrimp, firstly in the cornstarch, secondly the egg and finally the coconut.

3. Transfer the coated shrimp to the air fryer basket. 4. Repeat steps 2 and 3 until the basket has a layer of shrimp with room in between each. You may need to do the shrimp in stages.

5. Warm for 15 minutes at a temperature of 330°F and remove to enjoy hot.

Helpful Tips: You can use frozen shrimp in this recipe. Make sure that they are still cold but defrosted.

Crab Cakes

Total Prep & Cooking Time: 1 hour 20
minutes Makes: 6 Cakes Protein: 8 gm.

Net Carbs: 5 gm.

Fat: 5 gm.

Sugar: 1 gm.

Calories: 100

What you need:

two eggs, large

Dijon mustard - 1 tsp.

Worcestershire sauce - 2 tsp.

red bell pepper - 1/4 cup, diced finely

old bay seasoning - 1 tsp.

pepper - 1/4 tsp.

green onions - two,
chopped panko bread crumbs - 1/3
cup parsley - 2 tbsp., chopped
finely lump crab meat
- 16 oz.

mayonnaise - 2 tbsp.

Steps:

1. Chop the onions and bell pepper and set to the side. Finely mince the parsley and set aside as well.

2. Using a glass bowl, whip the eggs and blend the Worcestershire sauce, pepper, mayonnaise, mustard, and old bay seasoning until well-integrated.

3. Combine the chopped vegetables, breadcrumbs and parsley to the mixture until incorporated.

4. Finally, use a rubber scraper to combine the crab meat to the mixture and do not over mix.

5. Equally, divide the batter into 6 sections and create individual patties by hand.

6. Transfer to a plate and put a piece of plastic wrap on top.

7. Refrigerate for 60 minutes and remove when ready to cook.

8. Heat for 10 minutes at a temperature of 400°F.

9. Remove and enjoy immediately.

Fried Catfish

Total Prep & Cooking Time: 1 hour 20
minutes Makes: 4 Helpings Protein: 24 gm.

Net Carbs: 6 gm.

Fat: 26 gm.

Sugar: 1 gm.

Calories: 208

What you need:

4 catfish fillets
cooking spray (olive oil)
2 oz. seasoned fish fry or seafood breading mix 1
tbsp. parsley, chopped **Steps:**

1. Adjust the temperature of the air fryer to 400°F to heat. 2. Wash the catfish and use paper towels to remove the excess moisture.

3. Empty the seasoned breading mix into a ziplock bag and transfer one fish to the bag.

4. Agitate until the fish is completely covered, shake off the excess and transfer it to a plate. Repeat step 3 for the other pieces of catfish.

5. Transfer to the hot air fryer basket and coat with the cooking spray (olive oil). You will need to fry these in stages most likely according to the size of the catfish.

6. Fry for a total of 22 minutes, carefully turning the fish over at the halfway mark.

7. Remove the fish to a clean serving dish. Repeat steps 17 through 19 until all fish are completed.

8. Garnish with the chopped parsley before serving hot.

Helpful Tip: If you have a larger catfish, you will need to cook them in batches, perhaps even one at a time depending on the size of your air fryer. Feel free to add more seasoned breading mix to the bag as the fish will need to be completely covered. If you have a bigger fish, you will naturally need more breading. If you like less crispy breading, diminish the cooking time by 2 minutes.

———————

Herbed Turkey Breast

Total Prep & Cooking Time: 45 minutes Makes: 4 Helpings Protein: 32 gm.

Net Carbs: 3 gm.

Fat: 10 gm.

Sugar: 1 gm.

Calories: 226

What you need: mustard powder - 1 tsp. bone-in turkey breast - 20 oz. garlic - 3 tsp., minced rosemary seasoning - 1/2 tbsp. pepper - 3 tsp. olive oil - 2 tsp. lemon juice - 3 tsp. paprika seasoning - 1/8 tsp. salt - 1 tbsp. thyme seasoning- 1/2 tbsp.

Steps:

1. Heat the air fryer to the temperature of 350°F.

2. Whisk together the rosemary, mustard powder, salt, paprika, minced garlic, thyme, and pepper.

3. Combine the olive oil and lemon juice to the seasonings and integrate completely.

4. Use a pastry brush to apply the seasonings to the turkey breast.

5. Transfer to the hot basket of the air fryer with the side with the skin facing down.

6. Fry for half an hour and turn the turkey over. Continue to steam for another 20 minutes.

7. Check with a meat thermometer to ensure the turkey is at 165°F before removing from the air fryer.

8. Serve immediately and enjoy.

_____

Pork Chops

Total Prep & Cooking Time: 15 minutes

Makes: 4 Pork Chops

Protein: 24 grams

Net Carbs: 6 grams

Fat: 26 grams

Sugar: 1 gram

Calories: 192

What you need:

1 tsp. paprika

45oz. bone-in pork chops

1   tsp. onion powder

2tbsp. avocado oil 1
tsp. garlic powder
cooking spray (olive oil)

1tsp. salt

2   cloves garlic, minced**Steps:**

1. Heat the air fryer to the temperature of 350°F. Coat the basket with cooking spray.

2. Blend the onion powder, 1 teaspoon of the salt, paprika and garlic powder with a whisk.

3. Combine the avocado oil and minced garlic to the seasoning and apply with a pastry brush to the top and bottom of each of the pork chops.

4. Transfer the pork chops to the hot basket of the air fryer and fry for 5 minutes.

5. Flip the pork chops to the other side. Steam for another 5 minutes.

6. Remove and enjoy immediately.

_____

Ribeye Steak

Total Prep & Cooking Time: 35 minutes Makes: 2 Steaks Protein: 7 gm.

Net Carbs: 0 gm.

Fat: 4 gm.

Sugar: 2 gm.

Calories: 376

What you need:

2 8 oz. ribeye steak
pepper - 1/4 tsp. garlic - 2
tsp.,
minced olive oil - 1 tbsp.
salt - 3/4 tsp.
parsley - 2 tbsp., chopped
cooking spray (olive oil) **Steps:**

1. Whisk the pepper, parsley, olive oil, minced garlic, and salt until combined.

2. Apply to the entire ribeye steaks using a pastry brush and set aside for 15 minutes.

3. Apply the cooking spray to the basket of the air fryer and heat to the temperature of 400°F.

4. Transfer the prepped steaks to the basket, fry for 7 minutes, and then turn the steaks to the other side.

5. Fry for another 7 minutes and remove to a serving platter.

6. Check the internal temperature by using a thermometer and cooking to the desired temperature as seen below in the Helpful Tips.

7. Wait about 5 minutes before serving.

Helpful Tips: The cook time for the recipe is for a medium well steak. Diminish the time by 4 total minutes for medium rare and by 2 minutes if you prefer a medium steak. The temperatures for the level of cooked steak are as follows:

125°F - rare
135°F - medium rare
145°F - medium
150°F - medium well

Roast Beef

Total Prep & Cooking Time: 55
minutes Makes: 6 Helpings Protein:
25 gm.

Net Carbs: 0 gm.

Fat: 6 gm.

Sugar: 0 gm.

Calories: 320

What you need:

salt - 1
tsp. beef roast - 2
lb. olive oil - 1
tbsp.

rosemary seasoning - 1 tsp.

Steps:

1. Heat the air fryer to the temperature of 360°F.

2. Blend the rosemary, salt and olive oil on a plate.

3. Lay the beef into the seasoning and flip over to the other side to cover the meat fully.

4. Transfer the beef to the basket of the air fryer and steam for a total of 45 minutes.

5. Remove from the air fryer to a platter. Layer tin foil over the meat for about 10 minutes.

6. Take the tin foil off and serve while hot.

**Rotisserie Chicken**

Total Prep & Cooking Time: 1 hour 20 minutes Makes: 4 Helpings Protein: 22 gm.

Net Carbs: 2 gm.

Fat: 11 gm.

Sugar: 1 gm.

Calories: 296

What you need:

pepper - 1/4 tsp.

1 whole chicken, approximately 4 lbs.

red pepper flakes - 1/4 tsp.

butter - 2 tbsp.

salt - 3/4 tsp., separated thyme

seasoning - 1/4 tsp.

Steps:

1. Clean the chicken by removing the insides and remove the moisture by using several paper towels.

2. Blend the pepper, butter, red pepper flakes, 1/4 teaspoon of the salt and thyme in a small dish until totally combined. 3. Spoon the seasoned mixture in the middle of the meat and skin of the chicken on both sides of the breasts. 4. Apply pressure with your fingers to move the seasonings throughout the breasts.

5. Sprinkle the remaining 1/2 teaspoon of salt over the entire chicken.

6. Insert the wire basket inside your air fryer and transfer the entire chicken inside with the breast side down.

7. Heat for half an hour at a temperature of 365°F.

8. Carefully flip the chicken over using tongs and continue to cook for an additional half hour.

9. Remove the juicy roasted chicken to a plate and wait approximately ten minutes before slicing and serving.

Salmon Fillets

Total Prep & Cooking Time: 45
minutes Makes: 2 Fillets Protein: 22
gm.

Net Carbs: 0 gm.

Fat: 7 gm.

Sugar: 2 gm.

Calories: 150

What you need: garlic - 2 cloves,
minced rice wine vinegar - 3
tbsp. orange zest - 2 tsp.,
grated finely orange juice -
1/2 cup salmon fillets - 2 5
oz. soy sauce - 1/4 cup olive
oil - 3 tsp. salt - 1/2 tsp.
ginger - 1 tbsp.,
minced **Steps:**

1. Fully blend the ginger, orange zest, soy sauce, garlic, vinegar, orange juice, salt and olive oil in a glass dish.

2. Split the mixture in half and spoon half into a ziplock bag.

3. Transfer the salmon fillets to the ziplock bag and seal the bag.

4. Place the ziplock bag on the counter to marinate for half an hour.

5. After the time has lapsed, drain the salmon fillets extremely well.

6. Arrange the drained fillets in the basket of the air fryer and heat for 12 minutes at a temperature of 400°F. 7. Remove the salmon to a serving plate and empty the remaining marinade liquid over the plate.

8. Serve immediately and enjoy!

Shrimp Scampi

Total Prep & Cooking Time: 20
minutes Makes: 4 Helpings Protein:
16 gm.

Net Carbs: 2.3 gm.

Fat: 13 gm.

Sugar: 0 gm.

Calories: 191

What you need: lemon
     juice - 1 tbsp. shrimp - 16 oz., peeled and
          deveined

     garlic - 1 tbsp.,
     minced red pepper flakes
     2 tsp. chives seasoning - 1
     tbsp. butter - 4 tbsp.,
     salted basil - 2 tbsp.,
     chopped basil seasoning -
     1 tsp.
     chicken broth - 2 tbsp.

Steps:

1. Install a 7-inch baking pan into the air fryer basket. Adjust the temperature of the air fryer to 325°F for approximately 8 minutes.

2. While the air fryer is heating up, combine the red pepper flakes, garlic, lemon juice, and cold butter in a dish.

3. Once warmed, remove the baking pan with oven mitts and empty the contents of the bowl into the pan. Replace the pan into the basket and fry for 2 minutes at the same temperature.

4. Remove the hot pan and insert the chopped basil, chicken broth, chives, and shrimp. Blend to cover the shrimp completely in the liquid and seasonings.

5. Transfer the pan back to the air fryer basket and heat for another 5 minutes and gently shaking at the halfway mark.

6. Remove the pan to a wire rack for about 60 seconds after turning the shrimp to ensure they are totally covered in the sauce.

7. Distribute to serving dishes and garnish with the basil seasoning before serving.

Tilapia Fillets

Total Prep & Cooking Time: 10
minutes Makes: 2 helpings Protein: 23
gm.
Net Carbs: 0 gm.
Fat: 2 gm.
Sugar: 0 gm.
Calories: 112

What you need:

cooking spray (olive oil)
2 tilapia fillets
lemon pepper - 1/2 tsp.
butter - 3 tsp. salt - 1/4
tsp.
old bay seasoning - 1/2 tsp.

Steps:

1. Combine the salt, old bay seasoning, butter, and lemon pepper until blended.

2. Apply the seasonings to the top and bottom of the tilapia fillets with a pastry brush.

3. Coat the inside of the basket in the air fryer and transfer the fillets to the basket in a single layer.

4. Spray the fillets with the olive oil and warm at a temperature of 400°F for 7 minutes.

5. Before removing to a serving platter, make sure the fish is completely cooked by flaking easily with a fork.

6. Serve immediately and enjoy!

Carne Asada Mexican Taco Plate

Total Prep & Cooking Time: 35 minutes plus 3 hours to marinate Makes: 4 Helpings Protein: 23 gm.

Net Carbs: 2 gm.

Fat: 11 gm.

Sugar: 0 gm.

Calories: 190

What you need:

For the meat:

> 1 large yellow onion, sliced thinly

> *2* lbs. skirt steak, approximately ½-inch thick*For the marinade:*

lemon juice - 1/4
cup olive oil - 2 tbsp.

> 5 whole chipotle peppers
in adobo lime juice - 1/4 cup 2
pasilla peppers orange juice -
1/2 cup ground cumin
seasoning - 2 tsp. cilantro leaves
- 1
cup brown sugar - 2 tbsp.
salt - 3 tsp., separated

garlic - 1 clove, crushed
oregano seasoning - 2
tsp.

pepper - 1 tsp.

Steps:

1. Place the pasilla peppers over medium heat over your stove burner and turn with tongs until they turn black.

2. Turn the burner off and move the peppers to a paper towel to cool.

3. After approximately 5 minutes, use rubber gloves to remove the skins and set to the side.

4. Using a food blender, whisk the crushed garlic, ground cumin, cilantro leaves, salt, brown sugar, oregano, and pepper for about 10 seconds.

5. Combine the lemon juice, chipotle peppers, lime juice, charred pasilla peppers, orange juice and olive oil in the blender and pulse for an additional 30 seconds until fully incorporated.

6. Separate 1/2 cup of the marinade and empty into a separate dish.

7. In a lidded tub, transfer the remaining marinade and immerse the onions and skirt steak in the juice completely.

8. Refrigerate for 3 hours at least or overnight.

9. When the meat is properly marinated, heat the air fryer to the temperature of 400°F.

10. Remove the marinated meat from the fridge and thoroughly drain.

11. Transfer to the air fryer basket in one layer and steam for approximately 10 minutes, shaking the basket at the 5minute mark.

12. Remove the onions and meat from the basket and set on a plate for about 5 minutes.

13. Cut the steak into thin slices against the grain and cover the dish with the remaining marinade.

14. Serve with your favorite taco toppings.

Helpful tip: You can substitute jalapeno or poblano peppers in place of the pasilla peppers if you cannot find them.

Crab Rangoon

Total Prep & Cooking Time: 20 minutes

Makes: 4 Helpings, 4 pieces per Helping

Protein: 8 gm.

Net Carbs: 4 gm.

Fat: 4 gm.

Sugar: 6 gm.

Calories: 164

What you need:

> 3 1/2 tbsp. green onions, diced
>
> 1/2 tsp.
> Worcestershire sauce 4 oz. crab meat, finely diced salt - 1/8 tsp.
>
> 3 1/2 oz. cream cheese, softened
>
> 16 wonton wrappers
>
> 1/2 tbsp. olive

oil Water **Steps:**

1. Use a rubber spatula to cream the Worcestershire sauce, diced green onions, cream cheese, salt, and crab meat until incorporated fully.

2. Fill a small dish with water and keep handy.

3. Spoon the filling into the 16 individual wonton wrappers.

4. Dip your fingers into the water dish and run it on the edges of a wonton wrapper to wet them. Press the opposing edges together firmly on one side and then the other to finish with the pinched section on the top of the wrapper.

5. Repeat step 4 for all the wontons.

6. Apply the olive oil to the total wonton with a pastry brush.

7. Arrange the wontons in a single layer and allowing room to in between. You will most likely need to do these in stages.

8. Heat at a temperature of 360°F for approximately 6 minutes and remove to a serving plate.

9. Repeat steps 6 and 7 until all the wontons are complete.

10. Enjoy immediately.

Helpful Tip: You can substitute 8 egg roll wrappers for the wonton wrappers. Just cut them in half to be the correct size.

Total Prep & Cooking Time: 45
minutes Makes: 4 Helpings Protein:
4 gm.
Net Carbs: 28 gm.
Fat: 5 gm.

Sugar: 4 gm.

Calories: 190

What you need:

4 tbsp. olive oil, separated

3 cups green cabbage, shredded

1 clove garlic, grated

4 oz. red cabbage, shredded1 tsp. ginger, grated

4 oz. carrots, shredded

1 scallion, sliced thinly

3 tsp. lime juice

1/2 cup onions, diced

10 oz. medium shrimp

2 tsp. soy sauce

1 large egg white 8 egg roll wrappers 2 tbsp. water **Steps:**

1. Cover a flat sheet with baking lining and set to the side.

2. Warm 2 tbsp. of olive oil in a non-stick skillet and heat the shrimp while occasionally stirring until they turn pink throughout which should take about 2 minutes.

3. Remove the shrimp to a plate using a slotted spoon and let them rest for approximately 5 minutes.

4. Separate 8 whole shrimp and keep to the side. Chop the remaining shrimp into small sections.

5. Warm the remaining 2 tablespoons of olive oil for about 30 seconds using the same skillet.

6. Toss the diced onions and fry for approximately 3 minutes while occasionally stirring.

7. Then empty the ginger and garlic into the skillet and heat for an additional 60 seconds.

8. Combine the scallion, red and green cabbage, water and carrots into the skillet. Sauté for approximately 3 minutes and remove the skillet from the burner.

9. Blend the soy sauce, lime juice, and diced shrimp into the vegetable mixture until integrated fully.

10. Heat the air fryer to the temperature of 375°F.

11. In a small dish, whip the egg white and use the prepped sheet to place the egg rolls wrappers side by side. 12. Use a pastry brush to apply the egg to the edges of the wrappers.

13. Spoon about 1/2 cup of the vegetable mixture on the center base portion of the wrapper. Leave space on the edges where there is no filling.

14. Top with a whole shrimp and rotate the wrapper away from you while tucking in the sides to encase the filling fully.

15. Repeat for the other 7 egg rolls.

16. Completely cover the egg rolls with olive oil and transfer to the basket of the air fryer.

17. Fry for a total of 7 minutes while rolling them over halfway through the cook time.

18. Remove and enjoy while hot.

General Tso's Chicken

Total Prep & Cooking Time:
30 minutes Makes: 4 Helpings Protein: 9 gm.

Net Carbs: 23 gm.

Fat: 5 gm.

Sugar: 2 gm.

Calories: 430

What you need:

brown sugar - 3/4 cup chicken

thighs - 2 lbs., boneless and skinless potato
starch - 1/3 cup 3 green onions, chopped
sesame oil - 1 tsp. garlic - 2 tsp., minced
ginger - 1 tsp., minced chicken broth - 4 oz.
rice vinegar - 2 tbsp. olive oil - 1 tbsp. corn
starch - 2 tsp. cold water - 1/4 cup soy sauce
- 4 oz. 2 dried red chilies cooking spray
(olive oil) salt - 1/4 tsp.

Steps:

1. Heat the air fryer to the temperature of 400°F. Apply a coat of cooking spray on the inside of the air fryer basket. 2. Chop the meat into small chunks and toss in a glass dish with the potato starch to cover completely.

3. Transfer to the basket of the air fryer using tongs and steam for a total of approximately 25 minutes. Make sure to toss the basket about every 5 minutes to ensure they are properly cooked.

4. In the meantime, use a skillet to warm the olive oil for approximately 30 seconds.

5. Combine the garlic, dried chilies, ginger, and green onions in the skillet for about 60 seconds.

6. Then blend the chicken broth, rice vinegar, brown sugar, salt, and sesame oil into the hot skillet. Turn the heat up to simmer and occasionally blend for an additional 3 minutes while the mixture reduces.

7. Remove the chicken from the air fryer basket and transfer to the skillet. Stir to combine well.

8. Blend in the cold water and the cornstarch and stir for about 60 seconds while the sauce thickens.

9. Remove to a serving plate and enjoy!

Indian Paneer Pappad

Total Prep & Cooking Time: 20
minutes Makes: 4 Helpings Protein:
2 gm.

Net Carbs: 7 gm.

Fat: 0 gm.

Sugar: 0 gm.

Calories: 41

What you need:

 1/4 tsp. garam masala

 10 oz. paneer, thick and long slices

 1/2 tsp. red chili powder

 5 pappads, roasted

 1/4 cup water 4 oz. all-
purpose flour cooking spray
(olive oil) **Steps:**

1. Combine the chili powder, garam masala and paneer in a glass dish making sure the cheese is covered in the seasonings fully.

2. In a separate dish, blend the water and flour and on a plate, crush the pappads into small pieces.

3. Coat each slice of paneer in the flour and then roll in the pappad crumbs, completely covering the paneer.

4. Apply the olive oil spray to the top of the paneer sticks and transfer into the basket of the air fryer making sure there is room in between each piece.

5. Adjust the air fryer temperature to 360°F and heat for approximately 4 minutes.

6. Flip the paneer over to the other side and spray once again with the olive oil. Steam for another 3 minutes.

7. Serve immediately and enjoy while hot.

Indian Samosas

Total Prep & Cooking Time: 70 minutes
Makes: 5 Helpings, 2 Samosas per Helping
Protein: 6 gm.

Net Carbs: 12 gm.

Fat: 7 gm.

Sugar: 1 gm.

Calories: 84

What you need:

For the samosa breading: allpurpose
flour - 1 1/2 cups salt - 1/2
tsp.

thyme seasoning - 1 tsp.
water - 2/3 cup olive oil -
4 tbsp., separated *For the
filling:*

turmeric powder - 1/2 tsp.
coriander powder - 1 tsp. ginger
- 1/2 tsp., minced 3 russet
potatoes garlic - 1/2 tsp., minced
2 green chilies, chopped green
peas - 1/3 cup mustard seeds -
1/2 tsp. 4 curry leaves salt - 1 1/2
tsp., separated

1 large onion chili powder
- 3/4 tsp.

cumin powder - 1/2 tsp.

lemon juice - 3 tbsp. sesame
seeds - 1 tsp.

olive oil - 3 tbsp., separated garam
masala - 1/2 tsp.

water - 6 cups coriander - 2
tbsp., chopped **Steps:**

1. Peel the skins off the potatoes by using a vegetable peeler.
2. Warm the 6 cups of water in a saucepan with one teaspoon of the salt and bring to a simmer.

3. Lower the setting to medium, transfer the skinned potatoes to the pot and cover with a lid.

4. Bake the russet potatoes for approximately 15 minutes until they are tender and remove from the stove. 5. Thoroughly drain the water and crush the potatoes completely with a masher. Set to the side.

6. Dissolve 2 tbsps. of olive oil in a hot wok and toss in the curry leaves and mustard seeds.

7. After about half a minute, blend the ginger, chopped onions, and garlic before frying for approximately 2 minutes.

8. Combine the peas, green chilies, 1/2 teaspoon of the salt and chopped coriander and incorporate fully for about 30 seconds.

9. Blend the turmeric, chili powder, coriander powder, lemon juice, garam masala in the wok and sauté for an additional 2 minutes.

10. Fully incorporate the mashed potatoes in the wok, blending fully for another 3 minutes. Remove the filling from the burner.

11. In a food blender, whip the olive oil, salt, thyme and 1/2 cup of the water for approximately 2 minutes. The consistency will become thick dough.

12. Cover a dishcloth on top of the bowl and let it sit for 15 minutes.

13. Set a shallow dish out with the remaining 1/8 cup of water.

14. Section the dough in 10 equal sections. Flatten each section into rectangles about six inches wide and four inches tall with a rolling pin.

15. Heat the air fryer to the temperature of 360°F.

16. Slice the dough in diagonals to create 2 triangles. Spoon approximately 1 tablespoon of filling into one triangle and cover with the other triangle.

17. Dip your fingers in the dish of water and run on the edges of the dough.

18. Compress and crimp along the entire edge.

19. Repeat steps 15 through 17 for each of the samosas. 20. Use a pastry brush to completely cover the samosas in the last 2 tablespoons of oil and dust the tops with the sesame seeds.

21. Insert the samosas into the basket of the air fryer and steam for approximately 17 minutes.

22. Remove to a serving plate and enjoy immediately.

Mexican Churros

Total Prep & Cooking Time: 10 minutes

Makes: 8 Churros

Protein: 4 gm.

Net Carbs: 16 gm.

Fat: 3 gm.

Sugar: 6 gm.

Calories: 102

What you need:

1/2 cup all-purpose flour

1   8 oz. can refrigerated crescent rolls

2   tbsp. butter

1   tbsp. ground cinnamon

2 tbsp. sugar, granulated**Steps:**

1.   Use baking lining to cover a flat sheet and set to the side.

2. Dissolve the butter in a pot and take away from the burner. Set aside.

3. Heat the air fryer to the temperature of 330°F. 4. Blend the cinnamon and sugar in a glass dish with a whisk.

5. Evenly spread the flour on a flat surface and open the can of crescent rolls.

6. Flatten the 4 sections of rectangle dough onto the flour and compress the perforations in the dough to make one uniform piece.

7. Coat the melted butter onto the flattened dough. 8. Dust two of the pieces of dough with a tablespoon each of with the sugar mixture covering to the edges.

9. Place the additional pieces of dough on top of the sugar mixture with the buttered dough on the top and slightly press the edges.

10. Cut each section of dough into 4 equal strips with a knife or pizza cutter.

11. Rotate each strip of dough to create a twist and transfer to the hot basket of the air fryer in a single layer. 12. Broil for approximately 5 minutes and remove to the prepped flat sheet.

13. Apply the butter to the top of the churros and dust with a tablespoon of the sugar mixture.

14. Turn the churros over and apply the remaining butter and the last tablespoon of the sugar mixture, completely covering the churros.

15. Serve immediately and enjoy!

Mexican Corn on the Cob

Total Prep & Cooking Time: 20
minutes Makes: 4 Cobs Protein: 4
gm.

Net Carbs: 16 gm.

Fat: 3 gm.

Sugar: 6 gm.

Calories: 102

What you need:

>1/4 tsp. pepper
>
>4 pieces corn on the cob
>
>1/8 tsp. salt
>
>2 oz. feta cheese
>
>1/8 tsp. onion powder
>
>>1/4 tsp. chili powder **Steps:**

1. Shell the corn and clean thoroughly. Insert into the air fryer basket and heat for 10 minutes at a temperature of 390°F.

2. Open the lid and dust the corn with the feta cheese. Continue to fry for another 5 minutes.

3. Distribute the corn to a plate and dust with the chili powder, salt, onion powder, and pepper.

4. Serve immediately and enjoy!

Spicy Chicken Wontons

Total Prep & Cooking Time: 20
minutes Makes: 6 Helpings Protein:
9 gm.

Net Carbs: 10 gm.

Fat: 15 gm.

Sugar: 1 gm.

Calories: 192

What you need:

1 cup chicken, shredded

1 tbsp. buffalo sauce

1   scallion, green, sliced thinly 2   tbsp.
blue cheese, crumbled

        12 wonton
wrappers 1/8 cup water
cooking spray (olive oil)
    8 oz. cream cheese,
softened **Steps:**

1.   Cover the shredded chicken with the buffalo sauce in a glass dish and set to the side.

2.   Using a food blender, pulse the cream cheese, spiced chicken, scallion and blue cheese for approximately 60 seconds until combined.

3.   Heat the air fryer to the temperature of 400°F.

4.   Empty the water into a shallow dish.

5.   Lay the wonton wrappers side by side on the counter or baking sheet.

6.   Spoon about a tablespoon of the filling into each wrapper.

7.   Wet the edges of one wonton wrapper after you have dipped your fingers with the water.

8.   Crimp the opposing corners of the wrapper and then press the other opposing sides together to enclose the filling fully.

9.   Repeat steps 7 and 8 until all wontons are crimped. 10. Grease the basket with the cooking spray in addition to the base of each wonton.

11.   Arrange the wontons in the basket without touching each other.

12. Heat for approximately 4 minutes and remove to a serving plate.

13. Repeat steps 11 and 12 if it is necessary to fry in stages.

14. Enjoy immediately.

Helpful Tip: You can create the filling and refrigerate ahead of time. The mixture will keep for 7 days or will work as a dip at your next party.

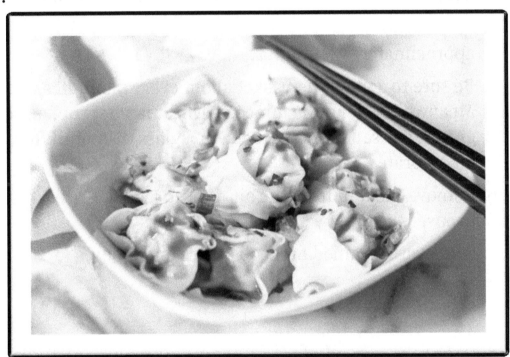

Sweet & Sour Tofu and Broccoli Meal

Total Prep & Cooking Time: 30
minutes Makes: 5 Helpings Protein:
4 gm.

Net Carbs: 16 gm.

Fat: 3 gm.

Sugar: 6 gm.

Calories: 102

What you need: maple

syrup - 2 tbsp. tofu -
16oz., extra firm 1 clove
garlic, minced soy sauce -
2 tbsp. ginger - 1 tsp.,
minced sriracha - 4 tbsp.

Steps:

1. Adjust the temperature of the air fryer to 400°F.

2. Drain the tofu and slice into cubes about half an inch wide.

3. Transfer to the basket of the air fryer and heat for approximately 15 minutes.

4. Be sure to agitate the basket about every 5 minutes. 5. Meanwhile, blend the minced garlic, maple syrup, minced ginger, soy sauce and sriracha in a glass dish until fully incorporated.

6. Remove the tofu from the air fryer to a dish, drizzle the sauce to cover the tofu by tossing completely.

7. Serve with steamed broccoli or rice and enjoy!

Tempeh Sandwich

Total Prep & Cooking Time: 1
hour Makes: 2 Sandwiches
Protein: 11 gm.
Net Carbs: 14 gm.
Fat: 4 gm.
Sugar: 4 gm.
Calories: 182

What you need: soy
sauce - 2 tbsp. garlic
powder - 1/2 tsp.
tempeh - 8 oz.

4 slices whole grain bread

4 tomato slices 4 lettuce
leaves liquid smoke -
1/2 tsp. rice vinegar - 1
tbsp.
ketchup - 3 tsp. 1 avocado
paprika seasoning - 1/2 tsp.

Steps:

1. Combine the rice vinegar, garlic powder, liquid smoke, soy sauce, ketchup and paprika in a zip lock bag. Seal tightly and shake to blend fully.

2. Cut the tempeh into thin strips and transfer to the ziplock bag.

3. Set the ziplock bag on the counter for at least 30 minutes to marinate or better overnight.

4. After the marinating is complete, drain the tempeh thoroughly and reserve the marinade for later.

5. Lay the tempeh in the basket of the air fryer and heat for approximately 14 minutes at a temperature of 325°F. 6. In the meantime, prepare the bread in the toaster if you wish and apply your favorite condiments.

7. Cut the avocado into wedges or mash if you prefer. 8. Remove the tempeh to one slice of the bread and drizzle the remaining marinade over the top.

9. Layer the tomatoes, lettuce, and avocado on top of the tempeh and finish with the last slice of bread.

10. Serve immediately and enjoy!

Apple Cake

Total Prep & Cooking Time: 25
minutes Makes: 2 Helpings Protein:
24 gm.

Net Carbs: 6 gm.

Fat: 26 gm.

Sugar: 1 gm.

Calories: 310

What you need: apple - 2 cups,
diced finely all-purpose flour -
5 tbsp. sugar - 2 tbsp.,
granulated ground cinnamon
- 1/2 tsp.

butter - 2 tbsp.

Steps:

1. Heat the air fryer to the temperature of 350°F.

2. Use a ramekin or baking pan to empty 2 cups of the diced apple.

3. In another dish, blend the sugar, cinnamon, flour, and butter until thoroughly combined.

4. Dust the top of the apples with the dry mixture and transfer the pan to the air fryer basket.

5. Fry for 15 minutes and remove to the counter.

6. Wait approximately 5 minutes before serving and enjoy!

Apple Dumplings

Total Prep & Cooking Time: 40
minutes Makes: 4 Helpings Protein:
24 gm.

Net Carbs: 6 gm.

Fat: 26 gm.

Sugar: 1 gm.

Calories: 192

What you need:

4 small apples

4 tbsp. raisins

2 tbsp. brown sugar

4 sheets puff pastry 4
tbsp. butter **Steps:**

1. Prepare a flat sheet covered with baking lining and set to the side.

2. Liquefy the butter in a hot pot and take away from the burner. Set aside.

3. Set the puff pastry sheets side by side on the prepped flat sheet.

4. Use a paring knife to peel the apples and then core. Transfer each apple to the middle of a puff pastry.

5. Heat the air fryer to the temperature of 360°F and line the basket with a layer of tin foil.

6. In a glass dish, integrate the brown sugar and raisins. Divide the mixture equally between the apples and pour into the core of each.

7. Enclose the apple fully with the puff pastry by folding around the apple.

8. Apply the cooled butter over the entire dumpling with a pastry brush and transfer to the hot air fryer with the folded edge down.

9. Fry the dumplings for a total of 25 minutes while flipping them over halfway through.

10. Remove to a serving dish and wait for approximately 10 minutes before serving.

Blackberry Cobbler

Total Prep & Cooking Time: 25
minutes Makes: 1 personal Cobbler

Protein: 3 gm.

Net Carbs: 22 gm.

Fat: 10 gm.

Sugar: 5 gm.

Calories: 200

What you need:

- 4 tbsp. butter
- 2 cups blackberries
- 1 cup all-purpose flour
- 1/2 tsp. vanilla extract
- 1 large egg
- 1/2 cup sugar, granulated

1 tsp. sugar, granulated and separate **Steps:**

1. Dissolve the butter in a pot and take away from the burner. Set to the side.

2. Heat the air fryer to the temperature of 350°F.

3. Use a 5-inch baking pan to empty the blackberries. Dust with 1/2 teaspoon of the sugar.

4. In a separate dish, blend the melted butter, vanilla extract, egg, flour and 1/2 cup of the sugar until fully together.

5. Spoon the batter on top of the blackberries and flatten with a rubber scraper or spoon to even the crust across the top of the whole pan.

6. Use a knife to puncture the crust in several areas and dust the top of the crust with the remaining 1/2 teaspoon of sugar.

7. Layer a piece of tin foil over the entire dish including the bottom. Slice a hole into the top of the foil and transfer to the hot air fryer basket.

8. Steam for 10 minutes and remove to the counter.

9. Take the tin foil off and serve immediately while hot.